Injury Prevention

AND MANAGEMENT FOR DANCERS

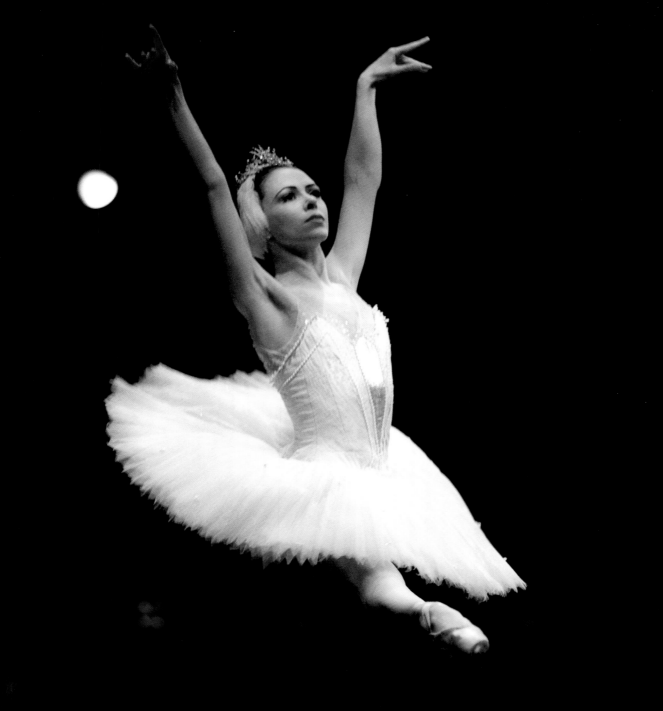

Injury Prevention

AND MANAGEMENT FOR DANCERS

Nick Allen

THE CROWOOD PRESS

First published in 2019 by
The Crowood Press Ltd
Ramsbury, Marlborough
Wiltshire SN8 2HR

enquiries@crowood.com

www.crowood.com

British Library Cataloguing-in-Publication Data
A catalogue record for this book is available from the British Library.

ISBN 978 1 78500 657 9

All dancer and exercise photographs by photographer Ty Singleton unless otherwise indicated.

All anatomical diagrams courtesy of Openstax unless otherwise indicated.

Typeset by Jean Cussons Typesetting, Diss, Norfolk

Printed and bound in India by Parksons Graphics

CONTENTS

INTRODUCTION

This book was commissioned to provide a resource for healthcare staff working in dance or with an interest in dance medicine. While dance medicine sits firmly under the umbrella of sports and exercise medicine, there are certain specificities relating to dance that may influence the outcomes with dance patients. This book is designed to give health-care practitioners a basic understanding of dance terminology, physiology and movement require-ments, and how these may relate to specific injuries sustained in dance. It will draw on experiences in both sports and dance medicine to propose models and structures of pathology-specific rehabilitation programmes, and will give usable examples based on dance patients.

When considering the rehabilitation of surgi-cal patients, it is important to discuss proposed protocols with the surgeon involved, to ensure they complement the surgical procedure undertaken and comply with any post-surgical restrictions. While the examples given in this book have been used with actual patients, it is important to clarify any rehabilitation programme with surgical colleagues in each case.

Furthermore, it is well understood that preven-tion is better than cure. This book will explore areas for general conditioning that may serve to enhance performance as well as reduce the risk of injury. The importance of the role of understanding the extent and nature of injury is also discussed. The need to create evidence within the healthcare practitioner's own environment is emphasized. Current thoughts on the structure and content of in-house injury audit programmes is also provided, to give healthcare practitioners the tools to support their own advances in the care of dance patients. Evidence-based infor-mation is a key driver within all areas of medicine and dance medicine is no different. This book draws upon the extensive research that has been published in the field (referenced in the Bibliography).

DANCE TERMINOLOGY

The assessment and successful management of dancers must reflect the specificity of their needs. This requires an understanding of the nature of movement and of the terminology used to describe movements that are specific to dance. The list of terms described below is by no means exhaustive. Much of the terminology is derived from the five standard positions used in ballet that relate to the position of the arms or legs.

THE FIVE POSITIONS

First Position

In first position, the arms are held in a 'circle posi-tion' to the front. The position will just engage the subacromial space, requiring the dancer to have good scapula stabilization, to allow for posterior tipping of the scapula, which will prevent subacro-mial impingement syndromes. The lower legs and the feet are held with heels together and turned out. This must be achieved from the hips rather than the lower leg, which would cause torsion through the knees and tibia. Moreover, it is important that it can be held without rolling in or pronation through the foot. Rolling or pronation of the foot may predispose the dancer to bone stress injuries of the navicular or tendon injuries to the tibialis posterior among others.

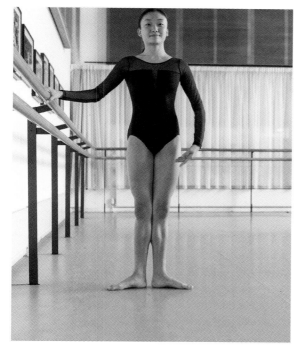

Photo 1   Dancer in first position with arms bras bas.

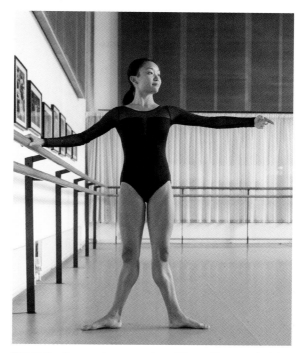

Photo 2   Dancer in second position with arms held in second.

Second Position

The arms are held in a rounded position with less than 90 degrees of abduction and in the transverse plane. Again, scapula stability is important, to reduce the risk of shoulder impingement. The legs are abducted to slightly greater than shoulder width apart and held in the turn-out position. Increased control from the hips is necessary to maintain the alignment of the knee over the (second) toe, to prevent pronation through the foot.

Third Position

In third position, the arm is held in first position while the other is held in second position. The leg corresponding to the first position arm is adducted so the foot crosses half in front of the other foot. This creates a smaller base of support. The dancer is still in a turned-out position, so control of pronation through good hip and gluteal activation is needed.

Fourth Position

From third position, the arm in first position is

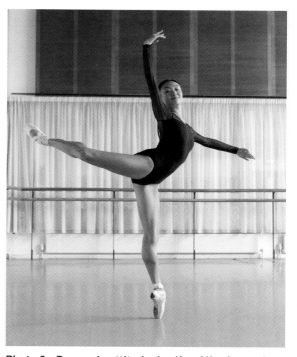

Photo 3   Dancer in attitude derrière éffacé en pointe with arms in fourth position.

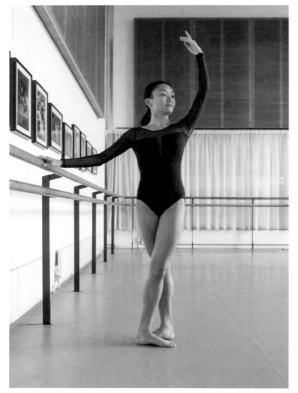

Photo 4 Dancer in fifth position at the barre with arms in fifth.

Plié

The plié is a fundamental movement performed to various ranges. Demi-plié can resemble a small knee bend or squat but starts with the dancer's legs in first position and heels kept close together and in contact with the floor. Failure to control this position from the hips results in rolling-in or pronation through the foot. The navicular drop has been associated with torsion through the knee, medial tibial stress syndrome, stressing of the navicular and increased pressure on the first metatarsal joint (made worse in the presence of a hallux valgus).

A grand plié can be performed from either second or third position of the legs and requires the dancer to go further into knee flexion. From second position the heels remain on the floor while in third position the heels rise from the floor, to accommodate the additional movement.

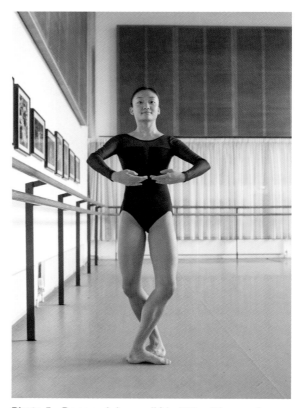

Photo 5 Dancer doing a plié in fifth with arms in first.

elevated while the front foot is moved forwards. Scapula stabilization is required through the range while the arm is elevated, ensuring good scapula-thoracic patterning.

Fifth Position

Both arms are elevated in this position, further increasing the need for good scapula stabilization. The front foot is adducted and fully crossed over the rear foot. This decreases the base of support and demands good gluteal activation in a tensioned and externally rotated position of the front leg.

FUNDAMENTAL MOVEMENTS

There are a number of fundamental movements that dancers will perform in class and choreography, which need to be understood.

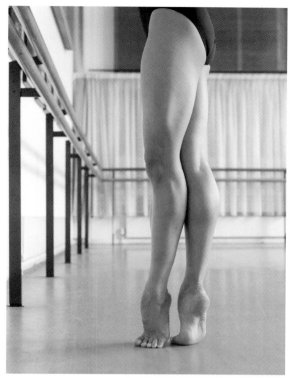

Photo 6   **Dancer relevéd up to demi-pointe in fifth position.**

Relevé

The term relevé derives from the French *relever*, which means to rise. The dancer performs heel rises, which may be from any of the starting positions to en demi-pointe (onto the metatarsolphalangeal joints (MTPJs)) or, in the case of the female dancers, to en pointe (weight-bearing through the tips of the toes). Most athletic pursuits recognize the need for good calf capacity, with the gastrocnemius and soleus being utilized to support the athlete. Good calf capacity is essential in dancers, so this must be properly assessed as part of performance evaluation or return to dance criteria, to ensure preservation of the forefoot joints. It is also important in the prevention of overuse injuries in areas such as the Achilles and tibialis posterior tendons.

Battements

Battements are dynamic, beating movements of the

legs at various angles. They may be tendus, with a small movement, or glissés, which encompasses a quicker movement, or grand battement, which is a quick movement from tendu and glissé to a higher position. In order to develop leg speed, it is important that dancers have good core control to prevent overloading of the lumbar region during higher movements. Failure to control the deceleration at the end of the movement can result in damage, either acutely or over time.

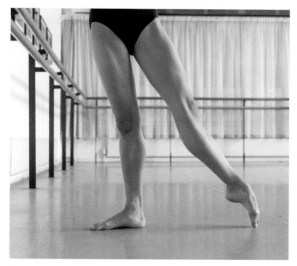

Photo 7   **Dancer performing tendu à la seconde.**

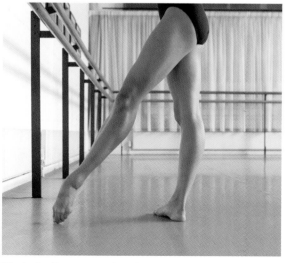

Photo 8   **Dancer performing tendu devant.**

Ports de Bras

Port de bras translates from the French as 'carriage of the arms'. Involving movement through the trunk into flexed and extended positions, it requires flexibility through the trunk and hamstrings. It is also necessary for the dancer to have good control of the core muscles of the trunk, to prevent excessive compressive forces through the lower spine, particularly with movements into extension. When dealing with patients with extension-related back pain, the practitioner needs to understand the technical capacity of the dancer's port de bras as a potential cause. Quality of lower lumbar movement may be compromised, with a stiff lower lumbar section seen and an excessive higher lumbar 'give' into extension as a focal point or hinge for movement, creating overloading.

Developpé and Arabesque

These are generally slow positions where the leg is 'unfolded' from the hip. The movement can be made to the front with hip flexion (devant), to the side into hip abduction (à la seconde), or back into hip extension (derrière), with either a bent leg (attitude) or straight leg (arabesque). The dancer must

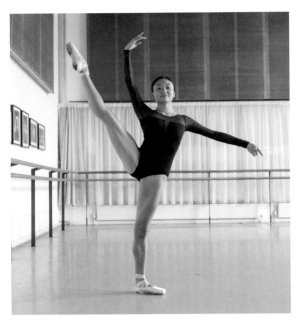

Photo 10   Dancer performing developpé à la seconde en face.

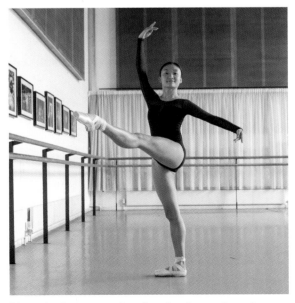

Photo 9   Dancer performing developpe devant en croisé.

maintain good alignment of the lumbar region and also needs to have the strength to hold the positions. Failure to control the neutral position of the lower lumbar region, due to less than optimal core control, can result in over-activity of the iliopsoas group as stabilizers, creating pressure on the lumbar region (and restricting the range of the hip). Movement through second position may create femoral acetabulum impingement potentials with cam or pincer morphologies. Failure to control movements may also result in excessive loading through the hip labrum, resulting in tears.

Arabesque movements range from small, with limited extension from the hip, to an extreme extension at the hip combined with some trunk flexion and extenuation through lumbar spine extension. Loading through the hip and lumbar spine needs to be controlled well to prevent injuries. In younger dancers, over-loading may manifest in stress response or stress fractures to the pars region.

Pointe Work

In pointe work, dancers (typically female) adopt an

**Photo 11   Dancer in
first arabesque.**

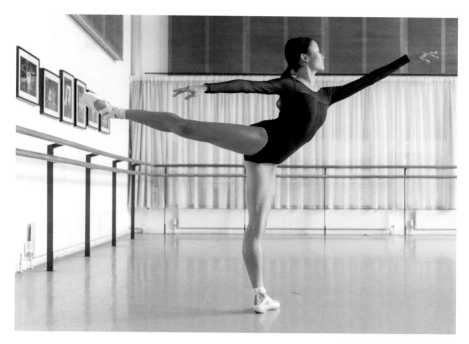

extreme position of the foot, weight-bearing through
the tips of their toes while wearing a pointe shoe.
Weight-bearing typically is through the first and
second toes. The shoe has a block and some arch
reinforcements to assist in supporting the foot.
Getting onto pointe may be a gradual process from
a neutral/flat position from the floor via a relevé, it
may involve a quick jump or sauté, or the dancer
may step onto pointe via a piqué. Whatever the
process, optimal whole-body biomechanics are
critical in preventing injuries when performing
pointe work.

Sickling through the foot can result in excessive
forces through the medial longitudinal arch. The
presence of a Morton's toe or hallux valgus can alter
forces through the foot and leg, resulting in injuries
if not well controlled. The flexor hallucis longus and
tibialis posterior play a pivotal role in achieving and
stabilizing this position. As such, they are at risk of
injury if they are insufficient for the loading required.
The alignment of the knee, hip and trunk all impact
on the transmission of forces. Over-extending when
en pointe (further into plantar flexion) can result in
posterior impingement of the ankle. The presence
of an os trigonum may exacerbate this.

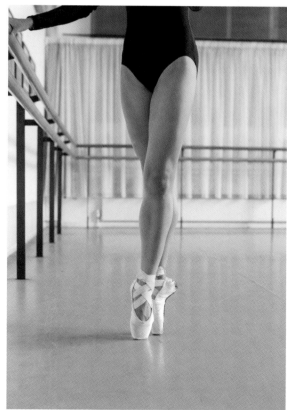

Photo 12   Dancer in fifth position en pointe.

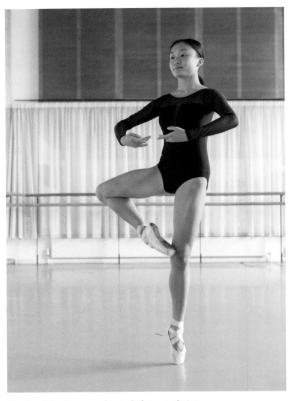

Photo 13   Dancer in retiré en pointe.

Turning/Pirouettes

When setting up to turn, whether performing fouettés or pirouettes, many dancers will start in a turned-out position of the hip. This leads to stressing of the medial foot, with increased pressure seen through the deltoid ligament complex and tibialis posterior. When turning en demi-pointe, the tibialis posterior is then required to stabilize the midfoot in a loaded position. Good ankle stability in a plantar flexed position is important. Turning requires dancers to have good trunk control and good scapula stability. To reduce the impact of motion sickness, dancers will 'spot'; this involves focusing on a particular spot and maintaining the head position until the spot disappears, then rapidly spinning the head round to find the spot again. Excessive forces through the neck are a consideration in this case.

Jeté

Dancing involves various types of jumping, using various starting positions. Jumps can be performed off both legs or one leg. A sissonné is a popular jump where dancers jump from two feet and split their legs like scissors.

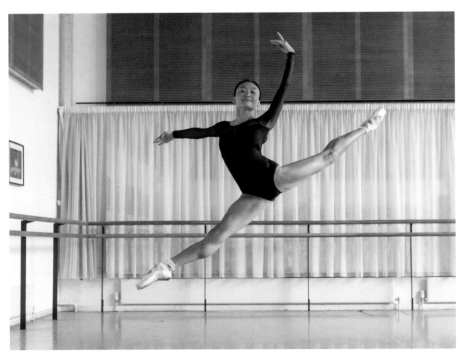

Photo 14   Dancer performing sissonné with arms in fourth position.

Jumping can be largely broken down into small (petits jetés), middle (jetés) and large (grands jetés). Smaller jumps see dancers using their lower leg muscles more, while larger jumps demand greater use of the upper legs and gluteal muscles. Strength, control and landing mechanics play a key role in injury prevention with larger jumps. Landing positions can be directed through choreography, so a dancer may be required to land in a turned-out position, increasing rotational torque pressure through the knee. This may increase the risk of anterior cruciate ligament (ACL) injury. Ankle sprains may also result from a failure to land correctly. More commonly in contemporary dance, some variations of jumps and landings (not always on the feet) can also increase the risk of other traumatic injuries.

Partnering/Pas de Deux

The nature of the dance style and the choreography may determine the nature of partnering. In ballroom, for example, it is typical for the male dancer to provide the lead. In ballet, the male lead supports the female lead to perform challenging positions or movements during a pas de deux, and is usually required to lift his partner. Lifting presents a number of challenges, with both partners needing to work with each other's movement and momentum in order to achieve the lift. A lift may extend to a full press above the head with one arm, which demands the appropriate strength combined with good technique.

The partner doing the lifting will be at risk of injury to shoulders and the spine, but lifting is not a passive process for the partner being lifted. Typically, but not exclusively, this will be a female dancer. While being lifted, a dancer needs to take care to maintain a good core and trunk position.

From a contemporary perspective, more movement-based descriptions may be encountered. While many movements have their origins in ballet, they have evolved and may no longer be easily described using the same terminology. For example, contemporary dance may involve more 'floor work', with dancers utilizing contact with the floor far more frequently than in ballet, and with 'crashing' to the floor not uncommon. This aspect of contemporary work can increase the prevalence of upper limb and even concussion injuries. Partnering in contemporary dance may also differ. Rather than executing some of the cleaner lines exhibited in ballet, contemporary dancers are known to engage in momentum-based lifts using rotation and angles. This enables them to create lifts where a smaller partner can execute a lift with a larger partner. While this may support artistic ambition, if it is not executed well, it will introduce a disproportionate load and an increased risk of injury.

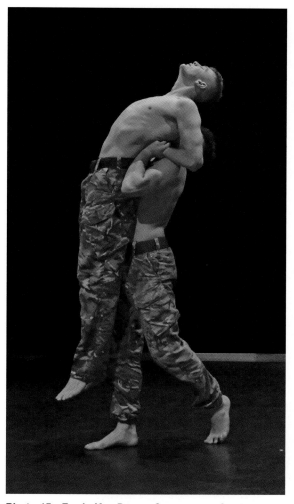

Photo 15   Rosie Kay Dance Company: *5 Soldiers.*
BRIAN SLATER

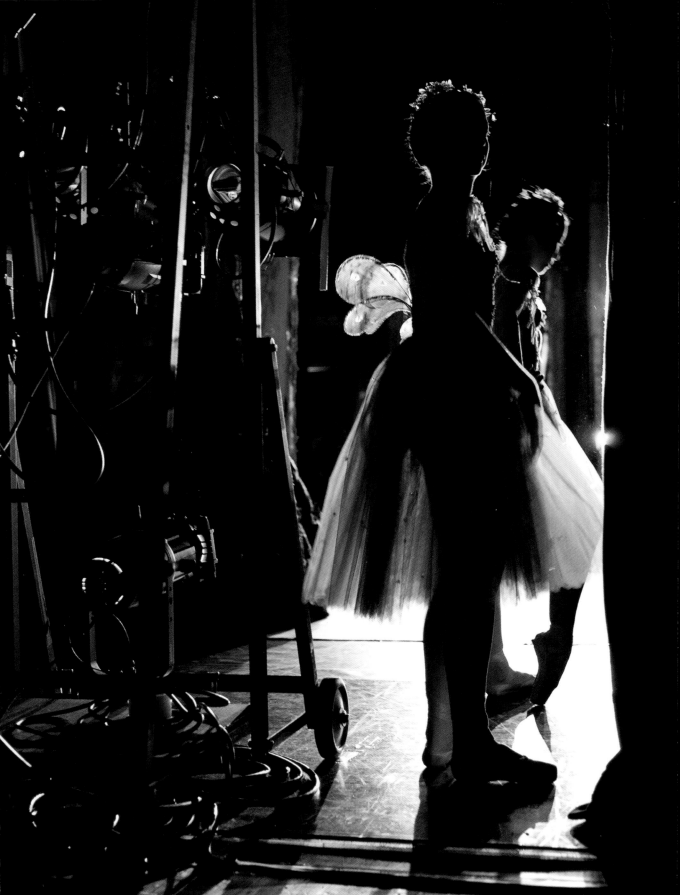

CHAPTER 1

BACKGROUND TO DANCE MEDICINE

Dance has played a vital role for thousands of years, as entertainment and as a means of expression in societies throughout the world. Records show various forms in India dating back as far as 6000 BCE, and, relatively more recent, there is evidence of dance being important in ancient Egypt and Classical Greece. 'Dance' is a generic term that covers a multitude of styles or genres. Classical ballet and contemporary or modern dance are the two dominant Western genres, but there are many other styles practised and performed in the UK today, including African, Ballroom, Bellydancing, Bharatha Natyam, Bodypopping, Breakdancing, Contact Improvization, Flamenco, Historical/Period, Irish, Kalari, Kathak, Jazz, Jive, Latin American, Line Dancing, National and Folk, Raqs Sharqi, Salsa, Square Dancing, Street Dance, Tango and Tap!

Dance is an aesthetic pursuit, with the cornerstone of many of the movements performed being derived from ballet technique. According to dancer, teacher and choreographer Anna Paskevska, 'Ballet is ultimately a logical technique; it favours the shortest, most efficient route from one position into another. This factor gives an aesthetic clarity to all motions.' But is dance a sport? 'Sport' can be defined as an activity that involves physical exertion and skill. Many definitions of sport go on to include the concept that the activity is governed by various sets of rules and can be competitive, involving a contest or game between two or more opponents. Given these definitions, dance may not be defined as a sport, but it is undoubtedly an athletic pursuit. Numerous studies into the physiological demands of dance attest to its demands for physical exertion and particular skills.

The benefits of exercise-related activities are numerous, wide-ranging and well publicized. They are physiological, enhancing health and preventing disease, and psychological, improving mood, self-esteem, psychomotor development, memory and calmness. The health benefits of dance as a physical activity have also been recognized. A dance-based programme may improve aerobic power, muscle endurance of the lower extremities, muscle strength of the lower extremities, flexibilities of the lower extremities, static balance, dynamic balance and agility, gait speed. It may also increase bone-mineral content in the lower body and the muscle power of the lower extremities, as well as reducing falls rate and risks to cardiovascular health. As such, the role of exercise, including dance, was the focus of a government initiative to improve the health of the UK through the Department of Health's 'Be Healthy, Be Active' programme in 2009.

PHYSIOLOGICAL DEMANDS AND THE IMPACT OF INJURY

The physiological demands and athletic loading in dance reinforce the need for sports medicine practitioners to be aware of the potential risks, and support these remarkable athletes. Additionally, the role of sports medicine is to protect and improve public health and fitness. While participation figures in dance may fall short of those of some of the popular sporting pursuits, it is a growing area of physical activity. This is most notable in young females, where there has been a concerning drop-off in levels of participation in sports. Providing appropriate support for dancers is, therefore, aligned with

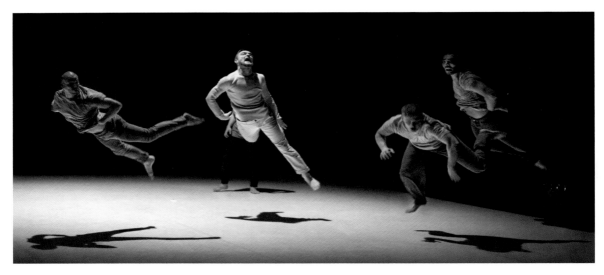

ABOVE: **Photo 16a   The physiological demands of dance are significant.** 2FACED DANCE COMPANY, **and** BELOW: **16b   Rosie Kay Dance Company.** BRIAN SLATER

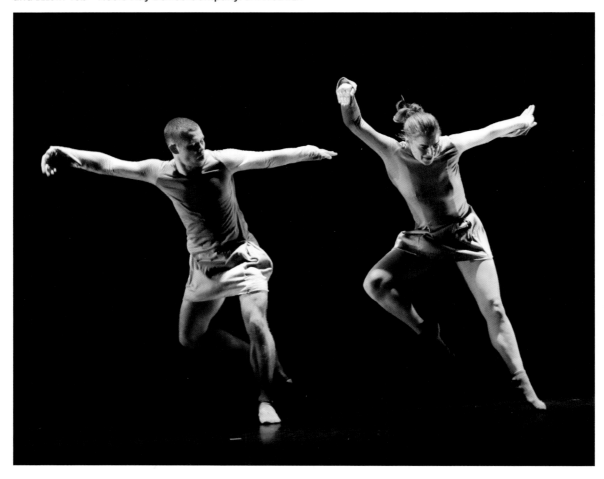

public health agenda. However, it is recognized that participation in sport or dance can introduce a risk injury. It has been estimated that the cost of athletic injury worldwide is around $1 billion, with around 29 million injuries (new and recurrent) each year in the UK. These injuries can result in time away from exercise and, therefore, less exposure to its associated health and psychological benefits. For non-professional athletes or dancers, the impact may extend to the workplace, with decreased productivity occurring through diminished capacity or complete absence as a result of injuries incurred. The financial impact will extend to costs to the National Health Service and any post-injury care needed for more serious injuries. Family and social life may also be disrupted by injuries, due to the limitations placed on injured participants.

The negative impacts of injury to elite, professional athletes and dancers can be significant. The financial ramifications of injury range from the costs of medical care to loss of personal income through withdrawal from competition or performance. The time away from training and competition can lead to a performance deficit, which could result in withdrawal from funded programmes and impact on the team or dance company's performance. Future contracts may also be adversely affected by injury history and status. The potential of a longer-term sequelae of injury also needs to be considered. In one study, eighty per cent of retired footballers indicated joint pain during at least one activity of daily living, and 32 to 49 per cent reported being diagnosed with osteoarthritis – a higher percentage than expected for their age equivalents in the general population.

Similar concerns over long-term effects have been raised in dance. Evidence of a higher prevalence of osteoarthritis in dancers compared with age-equivalent non-dancers was found in a study that measured radiographic findings of osteoarthrosis, including sclerosis, joint space narrowing, osteophytes, and subchondral cysts as part of the diagnostic criteria for osteoarthritis. It is noteworthy that the level of evidence of these studies is lower with some results from the reporting responses via questionnaires, and this may be limited due to a number of confounding variables and biases, including a bias in respondents who have experienced some of the musculoskeletal problems being questioned as well as other methodological challenges to high-level evidence. However, in the absence of stronger evidence to the contrary, it is reasonable to make a strong recommendation to pay more attention to the long-term sequelae of injury. Furthermore, reducing the injury burden on individuals, sports and dance organizations, as well as society, through an increased focus on the incidence and aetiology of injury and potential strategies for its prevention is surely to be advocated.

DEFINING INJURY RISK FACTORS

Injury management and prevention are a key responsibility of healthcare practitioners. Sporting risk factors have been defined by many authors. Hershman states that 'risk factors for a particular sport are derived by combining the epidemiology of injuries for a particular sport and the predisposing conditions that may lead to injury.' Although this provides a global view towards injury risk identification, there is a need to provide greater specificity to the predisposing conditions. Fuller and Drawer indicate where risk factors can be further delineated to allow a greater degree of specificity to the athlete and their needs; they define an injury risk factor as 'a condition, object or situation that may be a potential source of harm to people' and risk as 'the probability or likelihood that a risk factor will have an impact on these people'.

Risk factors can be categorized as intrinsic or extrinsic. Intrinsic factors are considered to be those specific to an individual participant, and can include age, strength and joint stability. Extrinsic factors arise from external sources, and may include surfaces, protective equipment and the laws of the game. Risk factors can also be divided into modifiable and non-modifiable. Modifiable risk factors, such as strength and flexibility, can be altered through training, whereas non-modifiable aspects, such as gender and age, may not be altered. Although the non-modifiable factors may not be altered, they can still be used to predict potential risk and mediate further injury.

One risk factor in dance that could be considered non-modifiable is the presence of benign hypermobility joint syndrome. It has been demonstrated that this disorder, which is often hereditary, is more prevalent in vocational ballet dancers and the lower ranks of professional ballet companies compared with a matched non-dancing population with an odds ratio of 11.0. Whilst there is no cure for this musculoskeletal disorder, which is associated with increased elasticity, an awareness of its presence allows measures to be taken to control factors that, in combination with the increased collagen elasticity, may predispose to injury.

THE AETIOLOGY OF INJURY

Understanding the aetiology (cause) of injury is a fundamental part of the healthcare process. Several aetiological models exist for injury in sports. Within these models there is an understanding of intrinsic factors such as age, gender, body composition, history of previous injury, physical fitness, anatomy and skill level (for example, sport-specific technique, postural stability), which may predispose an athlete to a particular injury. These, when combined with extrinsic factors such as human factors, protective and sports equipment and the environment, can create a susceptible athlete. The addition of an inciting event, such as joint motion, playing situation, training programme or match schedule, can result in injury.

In his theoretical model describing the causation of injury, Meeuwisse suggests that it is the intrinsic factors that predispose athletes to injury, but that they seldom lead to an injury on their own; it is the combination of both intrinsic and extrinsic factors that can leave an athlete susceptible to injury. Meeuwisse also indicates that 'an inciting event' provides the final variable in the injury causation model. Bahr and Holmes suggest expanding the model, arguing that the inciting event would often only constitute the mechanism of injury, but fail to document the

events leading up to the injury and suggest that this information can be more important in understanding causation. These earlier models have since been dismissed as linear paradigms that show a sequential event time line from the beginning point to an end point. The more recent models are more dynamic, allowing for a recursive nature of risk and causation to be considered. The recursive nature theory is based in part on the idea that the presence or occurrence of injury does not permanently remove the athlete from participation, and therefore does not represent a finite end point.

The original model by Meeuwisse provides an excellent foundation from which injury causation can be explored, and fits in well into stage 2 of the injury prevention model proposed by van Mechelen. The expansion of the inciting event by Bahr and Holme provided a further insight into the dynamic nature of injury causation, emphasizing that a multitude of risk factors may be involved, including, for example, a player's position within the playing area and their skill level, rather than simply biomechanical principles directly around the injury incident. While it is recognized that the key in injury causation may be the inciting event, influenced by the interaction of intrinsic and extrinsic factors, it is necessary to recognize the dynamic and variable nature of this interaction based on situational exposure. For example, changes in one extrinsic factor may lead to a different interaction with an intrinsic factor and result in the causation of a new/different injury.

One example of such an interaction in dance might involve the intrinsic factor of a lack of range of movement in the hip and ankle, and the extrinsic factor of the surface of the stage. A limited range of movement at the hips and ankles has been linked to injury in some sports. Specifically within dance, the presence of a limitation in the range of movement in the hip may predispose the dancer to injuries of the back, knee and lower extremities, including sartorial and piriformis tendonitis, anterior knee pain, patella femoral dysfunction, anterior impingement syndrome of the ankle, plantar fasciitis, and metatarsal stress fractures. A limitation of hip and ankle range of movement may also result in a restriction in jump height. A lack of range of movement, combined with a performance stage that has poorer force-reduction properties, may result in the dancer experiencing decreased ground reaction forces. In that instance, the possibility of injury will be reduced. However, where a dancer has more movement in the hip and ankle, allowing a greater jump height, that dancer may be more susceptible to the impact and increased ground reaction forces on a poor surface, resulting in an increased risk of injury.

The interaction of intrinsic and extrinsic factors may also be influenced by overall exposure. For example, dancers may be at the end of a touring period when they encounter a stage with poor force-reduction properties. In that case, fatigue may adversely affect a dancer's potential ability to withstand the new interaction of risk factors.

This is reflected in Bahr and Holme's example of an overuse injury and advice to allow for the longitudinal nature of the inciting event. The recursive model proposed by Meeuwisse et al. may facilitate better evaluation of this dynamic process as it allows for the athlete or dancer to continue within the exposure period and not necessarily be removed from the intrinsic/extrinsic interaction. Dr Tim Gabbatt, along with other research groups around the world, has extended the injury aetiological model even further by aligning the growing knowledge around the impact of workload with the injury sequelae. The application of aetiological factors to dance would include issues such as hypermobility within the 'Predisposed' category, stage and costumes under 'Susceptible', with 'Inciting events' including choreography etc. The understanding of this specificity in dance over sport may prove to be a tipping point in a clinician's success with dancer patient management.

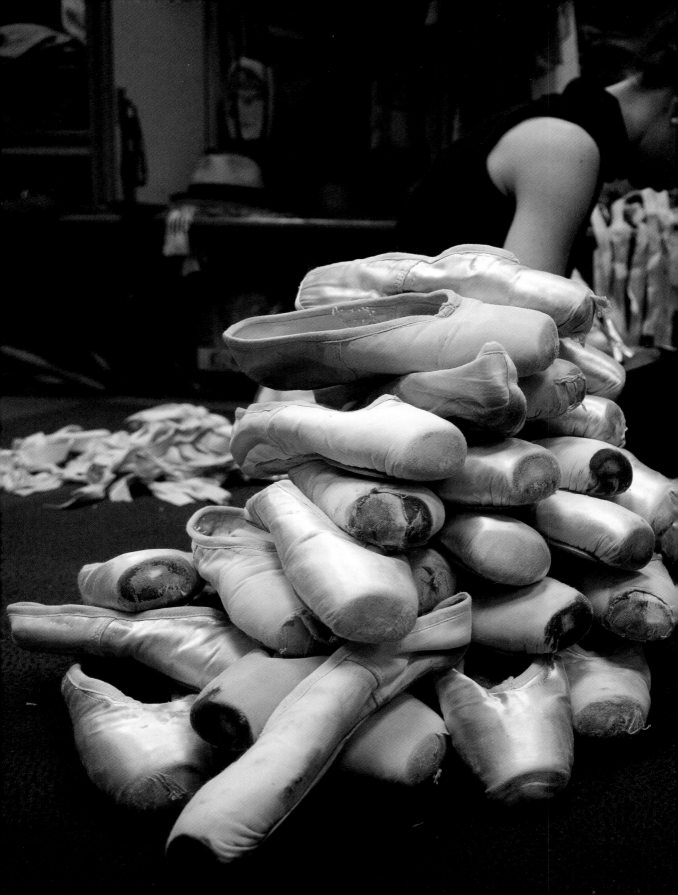

CHAPTER 2

CHALLENGES IN DANCE

While there are many similarities between sport and dance – even more so with certain aesthetically driven sports – there are also numerous differences. Understanding the specificity of dance may enhance outcomes, through an understanding of the various demands placed on dancers. This chapter aims to illustrate some of those demands and the challenges they present. It will draw from the aetiological models proposed by Meuwisse and Bahr and help develop an understanding of the extrinsic and intrinsic risks that are specific to dance. It will also help the attending clinician understand the terminology used in dance, to allow them to relate it to the physiological demands and the potential risk.

EXTRINSIC RISK FACTORS

Floor Structures and Surfaces

The correlation between playing surface and injury in sport is an evolving and developing area of injury prevention. Evidence suggests that a change in surface, such as a seasonal change in rugby or a move from hard courts to clay to grass in tennis, can have an impact on the participants. Dance is typically performed in theatres, but the nature of dance (particular contemporary) means that a variety of floor structures and surfaces may be encountered.

It has been suggested that the ideal force reduction properties for a dance floor should be about 60 per cent. For large companies, class and rehearsals

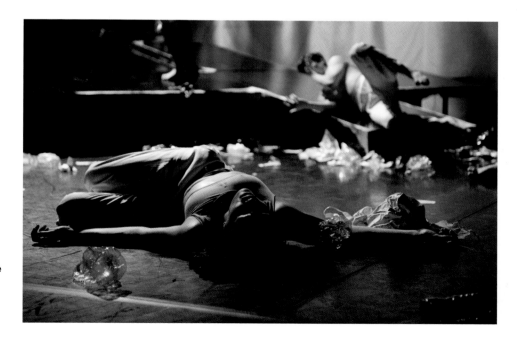

Photo 17 Rosie Kay Dance Company.
KATJA OGRIN

may take place in custom studios, but dancers who take class or rehearse in community-based halls are less likely to find a surface that demonstrates these properties. When it comes to performance, the stage of a larger theatre may not offer the optimal properties, either, with many designed to serve multiple uses. The floor may have been constructed to allow for a number of different types of performance, from opera to pantomime, as well as to accommodate a significant weight of scenery. The construction beneath the floor, with cross bridges, can alter energy return properties in different areas of the stage. As in a number of sports, consistency of surface can have an impact on injury in dance. The variation in energy return, from custom-made dance studios to multi-use theatres, to inconsistent areas in stage floors due to their very construction, is difficult to account for in preparing dancers.

The floor surface can also influence the risk of injury. Ballet is largely performed on a lino surface, but these can vary considerably in terms of their friction coefficient, which has an impact on the risk. This may be affected by the use of cleaning products or the transfer of oils (such as creams or massage oils) from the dancers' skin, which can create an inconsistent, slippery surfaces. Some dancers, particularly ballet, use rosin to help their pointe shoes to grip on a slippery surface.

These extrinsic factors serve to increase the risk of injury to dancers. Working with the industry, clinicians can look at stage and floor construction to reduce this risk. On an individual level, it is important to create elements of unanticipated control within training. Typically, dancers' movements are choreographed so that there are few or no unexpected movements. The use of reactionary drills as part of a proprioception programme will help support dancers in this area.

Costumes/Shoes

Dancers will typically undertake class and most rehearsals in tights/leotards or tracksuits with ballet flats, jazz or character shoes, or even trainers. When it comes to performance, their costume may be heavy or restrictive, or impede their vision (as in the

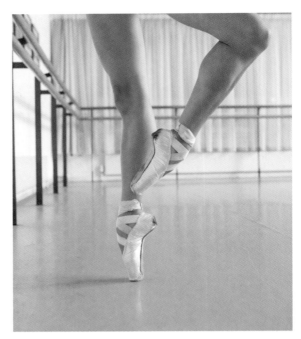

Photo 18   Cou de pied on pointe.

case of a mask or headpiece). Dancers will usually have dress rehearsals prior to performances, but these may only be in the immediate build-up to a show, reducing the training impact of working in their costume.

Footwear in dance may also differ considerably. In ballet, female dancers may be expected to dance en pointe, weight-bearing in pointe shoes through the tips of the first and second toes. For aesthetic reasons, some dancers may strive to create an extended longitudinal arch through the midfoot and increased plantar flexion through the talocrural joint. The impact on key areas such as the navicular and posterior talocrural joint is notable. A pointe shoe is designed to offer some support, but its construction is also driven by aesthetics. Some dancers will also 'break' their pointe shoes to help them achieve increased extension in the foot, and they may even use shoes that are too narrow, in pursuit of a certain aesthetic. In the presence of a Morton's neuroma, this needs to be considered carefully.

When not in pointe shoes, female dancers often wear ballet flats, as do male dancers. These offer very little, if any, structural support. Jazz shoes have some heel and forefoot soles, but little arch support, to allow dancers to achieve their aesthetic requirement of pointing the foot. Dancers may be expected to perform in character shoes, which vary considerably, from sandals to knee-length boots, and for contemporary dance, some performers may be barefoot while others may be in heavy boots. Female ballroom dancers often perform in positive heels while their male counterparts usually wear shoes that resemble jazz shoes, which offer some support but are designed to facilitate movement through the midfoot. All these types of footwear pose certain challenges in terms of injury risk.

Choreography/Scenery/Equipment/Lighting/Props

There is a wide variety of choreography and roles presented to dancers today, but along with that come numerous additional challenges that may have an impact on injury risk. For example, certain performances, particularly in the contemporary style, involve dancers performing at a height, which may see an increase in traumatic injuries. Due to the demands and costs associated with access to main theatre stages, most productions' rehearsals will take place in separate studio spaces. The studios rarely have the capacity to accommodate scenery and complete lighting, so dancers will rehearse with-

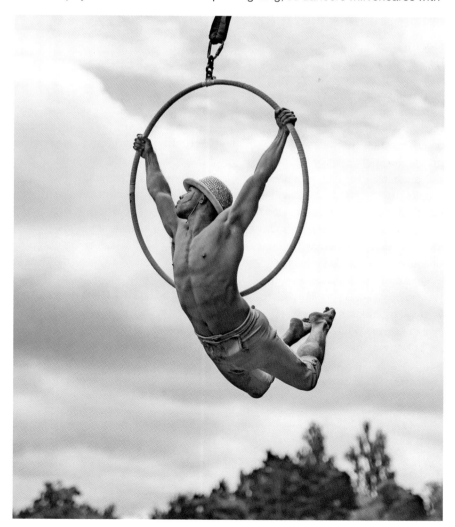

Photo 19   Demonstrating the aerial challenges in dance. 2FACED DANCE COMPANY

out these elements, but they will need to account for them during performances.

Typically, lighting in studios is very good. A particular level of lighting during a performance may be critical to the presentation, but it may also change the perspective of a dancer, being completely different from the set-up that the dancer has become accustomed to working with in rehearsals.

The use of props in certain choreographies, for example, swords in a production of *Romeo and Juliet*, will also present a challenge, requiring competency and skill acquisition if injury is to be avoided.

INTRINSIC RISK FACTORS

Training

Dance training is designed to support the highly skilled and efficient movement that is observed in professional dancers. The typical training for a professional ballet dancer starts in earnest at a vocational school, when a student enters what could be viewed as a full-time training position from the age of 11. However, many will have danced since the age of 3 or 4 years old in local dance schools. Kolokythas looked at the relative distribution of the different aspects of training undertaken at a vocational school. As can be seen throughout the dancer's development, dance-specific train-ing is the primary focus, becoming exponentially increased when scholastic commitments end at Year 14. Throughout the student's dance development, physical preparation may consist of only 1 to 3 hours per week.

It is important to understand the nature of the training and the development of a dancer and not to make assumptions around key physiological variables, such as strength and fitness, even for elite dancers.

The development and training process responsible for creating the efficient movement pattern, which makes the aesthetically pleasing movement with which dance is synonymous, may also create potential challenges for those looking to support dancers in their conditioning and rehabilitation. Dancers may not have been exposed to complementary training programmes, such as strength training, and work on core stability, which is more common in other sports. Time spent educating dancers on the objectives and expected positive outcomes can form an important part of the rehabilitation process, improving understanding and compliance. Part of that educational component may need to centre on expected aesthetic changes. It is not unusual for dancers to be resistant to strength training for fear of hypertrophy, or loss of flexibility. It is important that these areas are discussed to improve compliance. The lack of typical complementary training may also

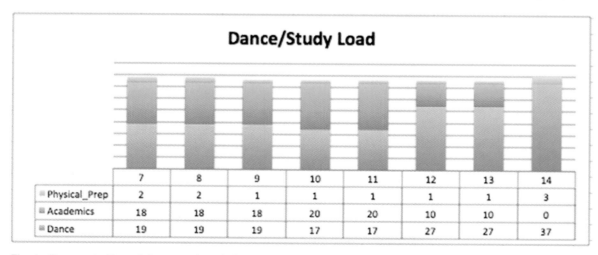

	7	8	9	10	11	12	13	14
Physical_Prep	2	2	1	1	1	1	1	3
Academics	18	18	18	20	20	10	10	0
Dance	19	19	19	17	17	27	27	37

Fig. 1   Demonstration of dance and study load in vocational dance school. (Kolokythas, 2017).

explain why research into various physiological variables, such as VO2(max) and strength, have demonstrated lower than expected results. Realizing the remarkable functional outputs required in dance, lessons can be learned from dance about how to achieve extraordinary outcomes through efficient biomechanics and movement patterns, despite the lower than expected physiological basis. It also means that there are new avenues to be explored in providing dancers with greater resilience against injury.

Workload

Large ballet companies tend to have a season that is similar to that of a premiership football or rugby team. It begins in August and runs until the start of the next summer. They may typically have a period

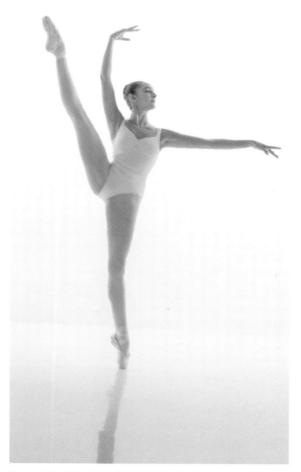

Photo 21 **Développé ecarté.** KIRSTY WALKER

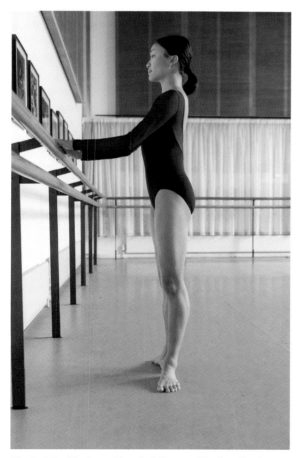

Photo 20 **First position holding and facing the barre.**

off (up to 5 weeks) during the summer, with a further week in the middle of the season. Smaller companies may have a less consistent timetable, and dancers may struggle more to plan their conditioning. Independent dancers who work from contract to contract are challenged further, as their financial situation may drive them to accept another contract in lieu of a recovery or training period.

A typical schedule in a large ballet company might entail undertaking class six days a week. Class may take around an hour to hour and a half. The format of class may vary but largely consists of three key areas: barre, centre and jumps. During barre, dancers will use the wall barre (and occasionally a free-

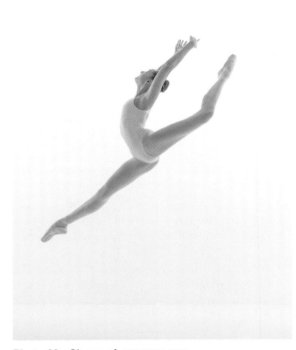

Photo 22 Sissonné. KIRSTY WALKER

standing portable version) to support and stabilize themselves as they undergo what may be described as a systematic warm-up and neuromuscular activation session, building up movement and intensity using balletic movements (such as pliés, relevés, and so on). During centre, they will no longer use the barre for support and begin to travel and turn. Finally, the class will progress to jumps, again incrementally, from petits jetés (small) to grand jetés (big).

Class serves to support and develop the technique and the efficiency of movement that are synonymous with dance. Through its incremental build-up, it can be used as a warm-up and to support strength and endurance.

Depending on the time of the season, class may be followed by up to six hours of rehearsals. A dance company may rehearse more than one piece at a time due to time constraints later in the season. If the company is large enough, they may have more than one cast for a show. Rehearsals will still take place during performance periods, although they will be reduced due to shows. A large-scale production may be performed between seven and nine shows a week, for periods that extend from weeks to months depending on contracts. A large-scale ballet company typically performs 150 shows a year. A West End or Broadway production may perform all year round and for many years, with the same dancers repeating the same movements week in, week out, year on year.

Depending on the size of the company and length of show, there may be multiple casts. If there is only one cast, there is significant pressure on each dancer, as they will be involved in all relevant rehearsals, as well as having the psychological strain of knowing that there is no replacement should they be unable to perform due to injury. The disadvantage of having multiple casts is that most of the work may be done with the first cast, with the result that the other casts do not have the same level of preparation.

Dancers may fulfil more than one role in a show, with some dancers undertaking numerous roles in a single performance. The variation in intensity

'RULE' CHANGES

Some sports have used the outcomes of epidemiological data to steer decisions around rule changes to reduce injury in their sports. For example, changing the start/tip-off in Australian Rules football has reduced the incidence of posterior cruciate ligament injuries, while rugby union is constantly examining the correlation between injuries and the scrum and contact areas. Those working in dance need to build epidemiological data to enhance choreographers' understanding of any potential correlations with their work, to support potential changes in order to reduce injury.

in workload and exposure may increase the risk of injury if the dancer is not prepared sufficiently. There may also be a variation in workload between different shows or choreographies.

Preparation

The better prepared a dancer is, the lower the risk of injury. The intensity and volume of the dance-related workload are an important consideration in the preparation for dancers, if they are to enhance performance and build resilience to injury.

Ballet dancers may attend class hours before a show, due to the nature of their rehearsal schedule during performance periods. Dancers supporting West End-type shows may undertake the Dance Captain's session prior to the show as part of their preparation for the performance.

An athlete will typically warm up immediately prior to competition, usually in the same kit in which they will then compete. Because of the costume, hair and make-up requirements for a performance, a dancer may need to undertake physical preparation earlier than expected or indicated. The timing of preparation for performances may also affect the timing of meals and nutritional support for performances. Dancers are often unable to eat at what might be considered an optimal time before a performance (3 hours pre-show), and, considering the dynamic nature of the movements required, may be reluctant to eat closer to a show when their schedule may allow. The use of home-made smoothies may be one way of providing the appropriate nutrients pre-performance that is better tolerated.

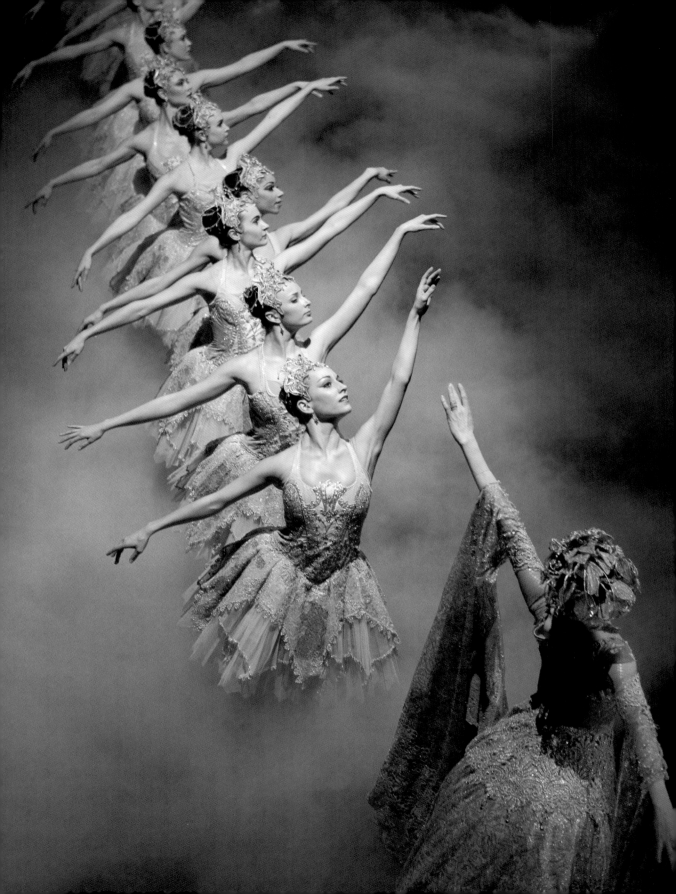

CHAPTER 3

INJURY AUDIT IN DANCE

This chapter will look to build on the developing understanding of dance through the aetiological models and the specificity of risk seen in dance. Aetiology is the branch of medicine that explores the risk of disease or, as in this case, injury. With a growing understanding of the physical and psychological impact of injury, there is an onus on practitioners to explore ways to reduce that impact on dancers, in the short term as well as the long term. In order to put in place a programme of injury prevention, it is important to be able to fully appreciate what injuries are occurring in a valid and reliable way. This involves extracting relevant information from aetiological models and applying it to an injury audit system. Knowledge gained from dance aetiological models should be applied to a programme that reflects best practice advocated in the current international consensus statements on injury audit data collection in football, rugby and tennis (in the absence of published international consensus in dance).

DANCE INJURY AND RISK

An understanding of the aetiological factors associated with injury becomes the foundation for any injury prevention strategy in dance. Further to this, it is essential to establish a clear model on which injury prevention can be based. At its foundation, the model proposed has the establishing of the extent of the injury problem, including numbers, incidence, time trends, severity and consequences, as well as the identification of the aetiology, risk factors and mechanism of injuries. This data is collected via injury surveillance or epidemiological studies.

The former is defined as the on-going collection of injury data; a number of approaches can be used, but the relevance of the data is largely influenced by the validity and reliability of the definitions of sports injury, severity and exposure. It is also recognized that, whilst it may be ideal to use the same systems of injury surveillance for all sports, the specificity of different sporting environments needs to be acknowledged and possibly reflected in the method adopted. This is supported by Hodgson-Phillips, who suggests that comparing injury statistics across sports may not be valid, due to the number of intervening variables. However, the more those variables are aligned, the more convergent the view that may be obtained both within a specific sport and across sports. As such, there has been an increased focus within sports epidemiological literature to both challenge and provide consensus statements to those methodological variables.

A consensus approach to injury surveillance will provide additional benefit for activities such as dance, which have not benefited from the same level of attention as better-funded sports such as football and the rugby codes, where more epidemiological studies have been undertaken. A number of larger national bodies have employed epidemiological studies as part of their accountability to their members and the organization, providing a valuable tool in determining patterns and trends specific to their needs and offering the capacity to interpret the results of any changes made. One of the longer-running studies evaluates the impact of injury in Australian Rules football, where, as a direct result of data collection, rule changes have been made. Re-evaluation following the changes has demonstrated a decrease in the original identified problem. At present there is no over-riding governing body for dance in the United Kingdom, with no long-term epidemiological studies being undertaken. The understanding and knowledge of injury incidences, and of the impact of those injuries on the United Kingdom dance community, are therefore limited.

While it is clear that injury surveillance and epidemiological studies can yield valuable information to aid the management and treatment of sports injuries, the validity and, therefore, the usefulness of the results are dependent on the use of an appropriate design and methodology. Consistency in study design and methodology can also enhance the ability to compare studies both within sports and between sports.

INJURY AUDIT DESIGN

Case Series or Cohort Design

There are two main approaches to injury audit design in sport. The first is case series design, in which injury-specific case findings, sport-specific case series or population- or institutional-based case series are analysed. The main issue with a case series study is that data collection is restricted to injured athletes and does not include information about non-injured athletes. This limits the ability to verify a study's conclusions. In addition, case series studies lack data on the exposure of the participants to injury.

The second method of study is a cohort design, which involves analysis between injured and non-injured athletes. Due to its analytical nature, it not only allows the measurement of injury rates, but also facilitates an estimation of the injury risk to be considered. The ability to differentiate between the characteristics of injured and non-injured athletes is a key benefit in cohort design studies as it allows a means by which assumptions over causative factors in injury may be tested. This may be of particular use in dance, to further develop the understanding of risk factors for this complex group of performance athletes.

Prospective or Retrospective Design

As part of the research design process, injury data may be collected retrospectively or prospectively. The use of retrospective design studies has been noted in dance. Major flaws can exist with the use of retrospective designs, including issues of recall bias and over- or under-estimation of exposure affecting the validity of the results. Gabbe, Finch, Bennel, et. al. (2003) indicated a failure in the ability of athletes to recall injury history over a 12-month period.

Using a prospective study design can improve both the validity and reliability of research findings, and therefore provide greater confidence in those findings, upon which interventional strategies may be based as part of the objective of reducing the impact of injuries. A further benefit of a prospective design is that it allows information from the aetiological model to be included in the injury audit collection, along with information around intrinsic risks, such as workload, recovery, and so on, and extrinsic risks, such as the surface type, footwear and props. Finally, an inciting event can be captured to understand the impact of the type of choreography and schedule, as well as the inciting event/mechanism of injury. All of these directly feed into a potential preventive programme.

INJURY DEFINITION

A key factor in the design of an injury surveillance or epidemiological study is the definitions used, because this will have a major impact on the nature, validity and comparability of the data collected. Within sports and dance epidemiology literature to date, a number of definitions have been used, as follows:

- physical damage via a sport- or dance-related incident, irrespective of its result in incapacitating the participant;
- injuries requiring hospital treatment;
- injuries requiring referral for treatment or medical attention/medical records;
- injuries resulting in a claim against an insurance policy;

- injuries that result in an inability to compete or practise as planned;
- injuries causing time loss from sports matches/ competition.

Although a number of factors may influence the choice of injury definition used, including funding and human resources, or accessibility to patient groups, it should be determined by the underlying objective of the research. For example, a study investigating the financial cost of injury may utilize insurance claims forms as an indicator of injury, while a study investigating the impact of sports injury on hospital services may utilize hospital attendance as an injury definition.

Although serving the purpose of answering the intended question of the researcher, there are limitations as to the external validity of some of the definitions. For example, the use of an injury definition that includes physical damage via a sport- or dance-related incident irrespective of its result in incapacitating the participant may not truly reflect the impact of the injury on performance. Similarly, there is the potential for over-reporting of incidents where patients utilize therapy services for maintenance purposes. In sports (or the few dance) organizations with 'free to the user' and accessible medical care in-house, this may be more prevalent. Such injuries would be difficult to document and classify for injury audit purposes, as well as analyse as part of a strategy to reduce the impact.

The use of attendance at hospitals or claims against insurance policies could result in an under-reporting of injuries, where only the more severe are documented. Similarly, the use of medical records could also result in some more minor injuries being missed, although they may still affect performance or contribute to the long-term sequelae of injury. This may be relevant in dance where medical provision for a large number of dancers is not always provided. As such, access to care might incur personal financial outlay, and dancers may choose not to report to medical personnel, opting instead to continue in an injured state or attempt self-management of their condition.

Some studies employ a time-loss definition, with only injuries that result in missing a planned session being recorded. It has been suggested that recording time loss from matches (in team sports) represents the cheapest, most functional, most accurate system, and the only one that can reliably capture 100 per cent or close to 100 per cent of the defined data. However, despite advocating this definition, Orchard and Hoskins, leading authors in sports epidemiology, indicate a number of limitations: it is less useful in sports where competition occurs rarely; a strong bias is seen against injury occurring in the last match of the season; the threshold for reporting is biased when matches may deviate from a standard schedule (for example, one game per week); some injuries are not identified through the use of analgesics/anaesthetics by players who choose to continue to perform; and there may be a failure to capture injuries that have a financial impact but may not result in a missed match. Further limitations of this system are that it may fail to capture those injuries that might play a relevant role in the sequelae of another (potentially more serious) injury and might have an impact on performance without any planned activities being missed.

The time-loss definition is clearly less appropriate in dance, where there is no uniform scheduling of competition. Dance performances may be sporadic or occur in performance blocks of 2 to 6 weeks, followed by a number of weeks in rehearsals. The use of missed performances may result in a large number of injuries being missed as they could have resolved within the time that has elapsed between performance periods. The nature of dance also means that, while a dancer may be unable to perform a more challenging role due to an injury, he or she may be able to undertake a less challenging one. Using the time-loss system, that particular injury would not be classified as such, although the dancer was unable to perform to their full capacity and undoubtedly had an injury.

Additionally, dance rehearsals may involve a risk of injury, with longer hours spent repeating movement sequences. Therefore, the rehearsal schedule needs to be accounted for within the overall understanding of injuries in dance. It is suggested that those studies that use an all-encompassing time-loss injury definition, which includes injuries causing time loss in training as well as missed matches, give a true global picture of injury incidence in sport. Reporting reliability can be difficult, however.

Using restricted activity definitions, the distinction between partial and complete restrictions is not always made, which may result in the seriousness of the injury not being fully appreciated, although this can be partially overcome by reporting injury severity. Using a time-loss injury definition in dance that accounts for restricted activities provides an opportunity to explore those injuries that affect performance. As such, it can have consequence for all stakeholders as well as providing a basis for strategic planning for a company wishing to invest in their dancers' health and well-being. Capturing data on injuries that result in complete absence from dance activities as well as restricted activities could offer an even greater understanding of the impact of injuries on performance.

Consensus statements on injury definitions have been published for football, rugby union and tennis. Injury definitions have ranged from physical complaints and exceeding the body's functional integrity to medical attention and time loss in football and rugby. The statement relating to tennis expands the injury definition into 'medical conditions' to include both illness and psychological aspects as well as injury. The value of a consensus statement derives from the process of key researchers and clinicians within the field discussing and agreeing on the best process for the development of epidemiological data. It offers a template on which other researchers may base their work, allowing a greater possibility for cross-study comparisons.

This process of reaching (and using) consensus definitions has also been recognized in dance. As the tennis consensus statement indicates, there is a need to both adopt and utilize aspects of the established consensus documents that have been able to demonstrate the value to this process in assimilating valuable data for their disciplines, but there is also a need to incorporate more specific aspects that would have more direct relevance to that particular sport/activity. The nature of the non-competitive environment in dance, which differs from those sports in which performances are objectively measured by times, heights, points and goals, could mean that a dancer can alter or reduce their maximum performance capacity to accommodate an injury and yet continue to perform. As such, it is imperative within the dance environment that an all-encompassing time-loss injury definition is used, so that those injuries that can affect performance but not necessarily result in full withdrawal from dance-related activities may be accounted for.

DATA COLLECTION AND REPORTING

Further influence on the validity of results of injury surveillance studies stems from the method of reporting. The three most common ways of reporting injuries are by using absolute injury numbers, the proportion of injuries and the injury incidence. Results presented as numbers or proportions offer limited value, due to the exclusion of exposure data – it is not possible to ascertain activity periods/exposure, when athletes may be at risk of injury – so they cannot be compared usefully with others. Using incidence, however, as a mathematical and epidemiological concept, allows for the inclusion of a defined population at risk as well as the time at risk.

Even with exposure recorded, the number of ways in which incidence can be expressed can challenge inter-study comparisons. Common methods for displaying incidence with exposure includes injuries/1000 player hours of exposure, injuries/1000 athlete exposures and injuries/1000 match hours. Expressing injury incidence as a component of 1000 hours of exposure allows for cross-comparison with other recognized sports epidemiological data, as well as leading to a better understanding of potential risk. In determining potential risk within dance, the need to account for exposure is critical, as there is a potential for dancers to undertake lengthy or prolonged periods of dance-related activities.

It is recognized that the literature on injuries in dance is weakened by inconsistent exposure techniques. Exposure can be expressed by two means: activity-based units, also known as athletic exposures (AE), or time-based units. The use of athletic exposures, where 1AE is calculated as participation in one practice or competition session, has been used by the National Collegiate Athletic Association Injury Surveillance Systems in reporting over a number of sports. However, there is a major limitation to its use as a measurement of exposure: the variation in time that each session may take. Competition in sport may vary from as little as 10 seconds (as in track athletes) to as long as a number of days (as in test cricket). Similarly, training session times may be very different. These variations make cross-comparisons between sports invalid.

Exposure may also be captured using time-based units. This allows for greater understanding as to the level of exposure that athletes have had and as such may provide a better insight when predicting risk. In dance, due to variations in length of rehearsals, dance class and performances, calculating exposure as a component of time (using a ratio per 1000 hours) would be more sensitive.

A limitation of both systems is that they fail to incorporate the intensity of the exposure session.

THE DISTRIBUTION, NATURE AND CODING OF INJURIES

The use of standardized diagnosis coding systems can improve inter-tester reliability as well as reduce the subjectivity. The Orchard Codes System is one system that is used within sports-injury studies. The need for coding of injuries in dance has been recognized. Using an internationally recognized coding system can improve both the cross-comparability of data and the reliability of outcomes.

It is recognized that dance may present certain challenges to measuring exposure, as the nature of different dance-related activities can vary with regard to energy exposure. Although individually calculated exposures for dancers would be ideal, it is recognized that, in large ballet companies, recording individual dancers' schedules of rehearsals and performances may be too time-consuming. In this case, average exposure calculation based on group data is an acceptable method. While the measurement of energy exposure during dance-related activities would provide an even greater understanding of the exposure, and subsequent risk to a dancer, its use during longitudinal epidemiological studies has substantial practical issues making its incorporation problematic and potentially prohibitive. Information related to the training load, even if only through a self-reported 'rate of perceived exertion', can add an important component to an assessment of the risk of injury.

REPORTING THE SEVERITY OF INJURIES

Both the severity and incidence of injuries sustained constitute key parameters in epidemiological studies, allowing the identification of the magnitude of an injury problem in a specific population group, as well as a consideration of intra- and inter-sport comparisons of the data. It also enables the relationship between risk and injury to be considered and provides the evidence to assess the effectiveness of implemented interventional strategies. Dr Brooks and Prof Fuller reflect this importance of injury definition and severity, indicating that the variations often challenge any validity of inter-study comparisons. The inclusion of injury distribution and nature can provide further data that will contribute to an overall risk analysis. Recording severity in dance studies is paramount as the potential for higher rates of more minor injuries might mislead healthcare providers when they are identifying the relative risks associated in dance.

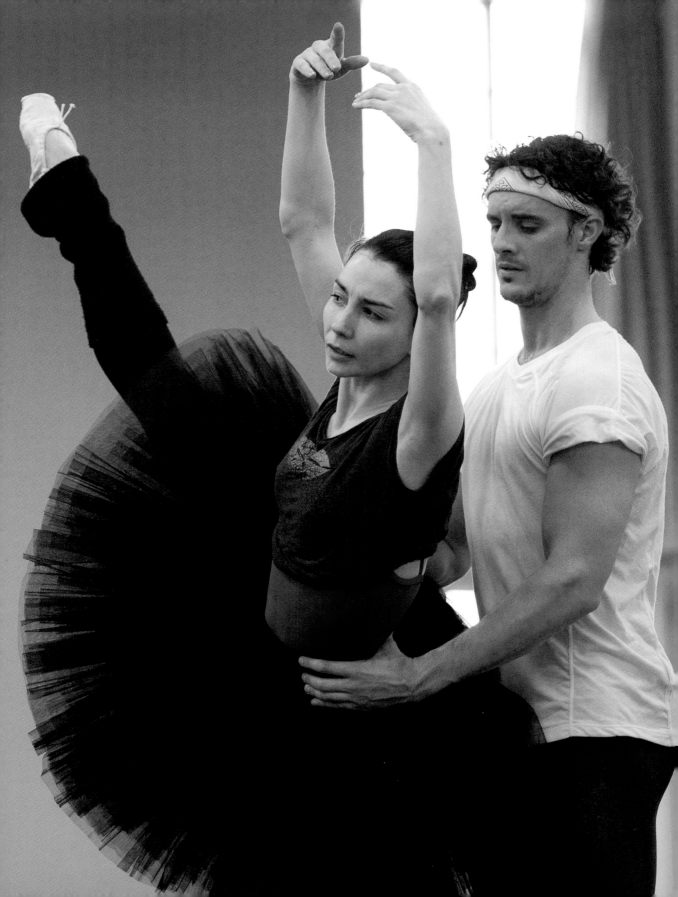

CHAPTER 4

PHYSICAL PREPARATION IN DANCE

Various procedures may be used to support the physiological demands placed on dancers. This chapter will introduce the concept of 'strength and conditioning' in dance as a broad concept encompassing all aspects of physical preparation. It will build on traditional routines often employed by dancers in their physical preparation, such as Pilates, and extend that to include movement competency, strength, power, muscle endurance and fitness. It will also touch upon the need to fuel and recover as key parts of the overall physical preparation for dance. It will go on to explore ways in which dancers can support and enhance their performance capacity through the application of strength and conditioning, with some practical programmes offered as a means of example and reference points.

INTRODUCTION

In most sports, complementary training is part of the overall curriculum. However, this is not necessarily the case in dance, and not all dancers experience structured complementary training as part of their development. As such, the term 'strength and conditioning' might ring alarm bells, evoking an image of gym-based resistance or weight training. The English Institute of Sport (EIS) defines strength and conditioning as 'the physical and physiological development of athletes for elite sport performances'. According to the EIS, its role is 'to use exercise prescription specifically to improve performance in athletic competition... [and to] help athletes with injury prevention and proper mechanics within their sports performances'.

Strength and conditioning can also be used to develop robustness in areas of the body not fully supported by the nature of the athletic discipline. For example, it has been demonstrated that resistance training can improve bone mineral density, with studies of elite female rowers demonstrating above-average bone mineral density of the lumbar spine. Dancers have been known to demonstrate lower-than-average bone mineral density scores of the lumbar spine, so complementary training – in the form of a rowing ergometer – would certainly be beneficial.

Strength and conditioning is not limited to working with weights or machines in a gym. It encompasses all aspects of physiological enhancement, including cardiovascular fitness, movement competency and plyometric training. This may occur in a gym setting but may also include work done in the studio. Dance is a discipline built on a foundation of technical ability and skill. The role of strength and conditioning in dance is to support and enhance this technical ability. Furthermore, research has demonstrated that a fitter dancer is rated as an aesthetically 'better' dancer by artistic directors. Training can also be directed towards reducing the impact of physiological fatigue on performance, with the associated improvements in resilience against psychological fatigue. Appropriate strength and conditioning can enable dancers to fulfil their artistic aptitude. As is the case with supporting sporting athletes, there needs to be a clear functional relationship between the exercise prescription and the desired outcome – typically, a particular aspect of the dance performance.

CONDITIONING FOR DANCE

Core Stability

Core stability has been a mainstay of the fitness and healthcare armoury for many years. Traditionally, a programme should include exercises that activate the 'core cylinder' of multifidus, transverse abdominis and the oblique abdominals. There are, however, a multitude of definitions and terminology in relation to core stability exercises, based on the different classification systems described in the literature. The more frequently utilized classifications of muscular systems include Janda and Sahrmann's system of stabilizers and mobilizers and Bergmark's local and global muscle stability system. As noted by Commerford, these systems are better linked when it comes to appreciating their clinical value. Given our understanding of the impact of functional instability due to 'muscle imbalance' and compensatory 'give' or failure to achieve segmental control during movement, Commerford's delineation from core stability to motor control stability as it applied to any region of the body is more applicable. While these may be key when considering a rehabilitation programme, the same principles apply when designing a conditioning programme for dancers. Core stability, motor control stability or neuromuscular facilitation provide the foundation upon which normal movement is based and create a safe environment on which higher-intensity exercise can be based. Without an appropriate foundation, higher-level exercise may increase injury risk. Furthermore, the right foundation allows for the movement quality that is synonymous with dance – fluid and effortless without compensation.

A good foundation can be achieved in many ways, including Pilates, Gyrotonic, Swiss ball, mat-based exercises and more recently suspension cable training. Each discipline has both strengths and weaknesses. Utilizing a cross-section of these core-based neuromuscular exercises offers a balance of training. When used correctly, they can provide an effective means to challenge and develop the control needed for the same achievement of a foundation for a dancer's functional requirements.

The development of a stability programme for dance can focus on key areas of stability, including the ankle, lumbo-pelvic, scapular and neck. In areas such as the hip and shoulder, stability and movement dissociation are key and these must therefore be the primary focus of a stability programme. Dissociation is also important in the thoracic and lumbar regions.

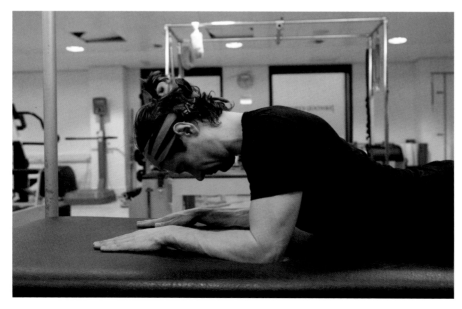

Photo 23 Start position for deep neck stabilizers.

Photo 24 Finish position for deep neck stabilizers.

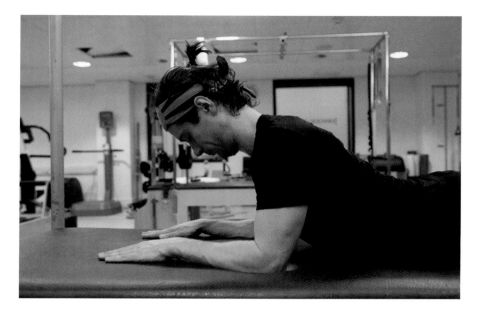

Photo 25 Standing position for deep neck stabilizers.

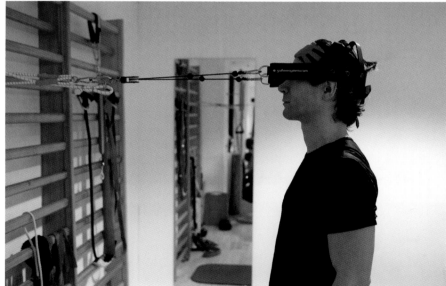

One key area of stability and control for dancers comes from the deep neck flexor as an important foundation exercise for establishing head control (Photos 23 and 24.). This is then further extended to introducing isometric control of the head in standing (Photo 25). Finally, a progression of 'spotting' is used to establish control through the range of movement (Photo 26).

Again, the functional requirements in pirouettes and turning demand stability in the thoracic region, as well as scapular control. Scapular control with shoulder dissociation can be started in a prone position (Photos 27 and 28) and progressed to standing (Photos 29–32).

Isometric rotational control of the thoracic spine is a useful way to establish this control alongside scapular stabilizing exercises (Photos 33–36).

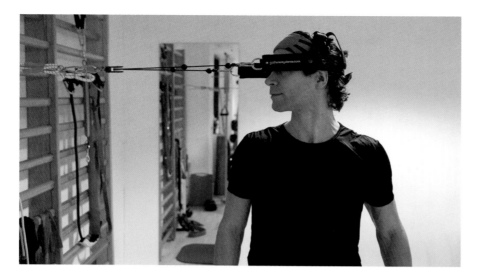

Photo 26 Spotting position for deep neck stabilizers.

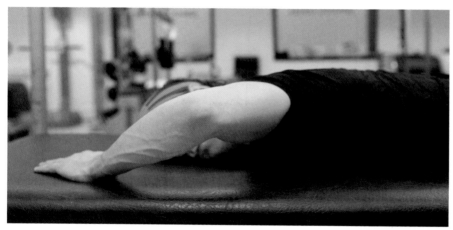

Photo 27 Scapula stabilization with prone elbow lift.

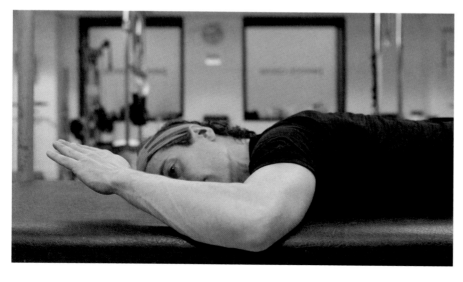

Photo 28 Scapula stabilization with prone wrist lift.

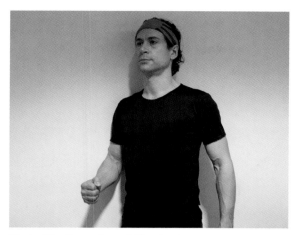

Photo 29   Scapula stabilization in standing starting position.

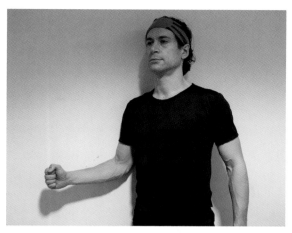

Photo 30   Scapula stabilization in standing finishing position.

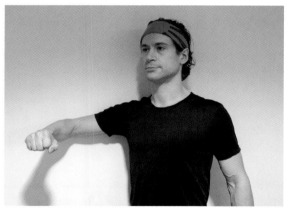

Photo 31   Scapula stabilization in standing and abduction starting position.

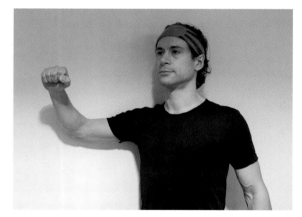

Photo 32   Scapula stabilization in standing and abduction finishing position.

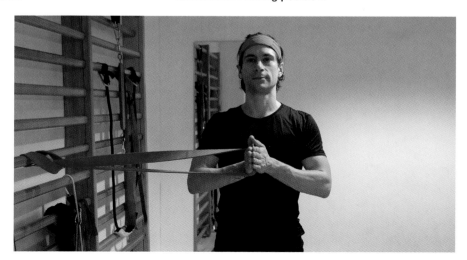

Photo 33   Palof press: thoracic stabilization in standing starting position.

Maintaining a neutral trunk position (both thoracic and lumber) is a key objective in movement competency drills. These can be combined with either scapular control with suspension cable reachers (Photos 37 and 38) or with a Swiss ball and hip movements like the Swiss ball sprinter's drill (Photos 39–41).

Hip dissociation and firing are critical to the overall stability required by dancers. Dissociation drills can start in supine with bent-knee falls outs (Photos

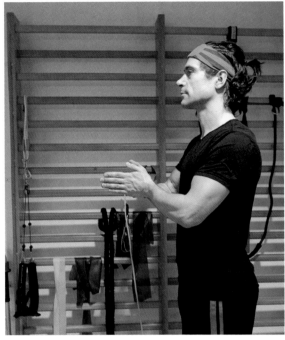

Photo 34   Palof press: thoracic stabilization in standing starting position.

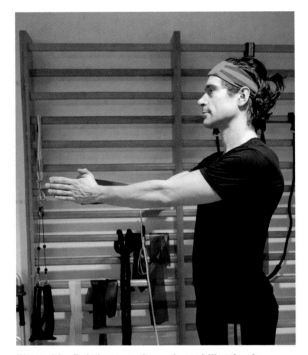

Photo 36   Palof press: thoracic stabilization in standing finishing position.

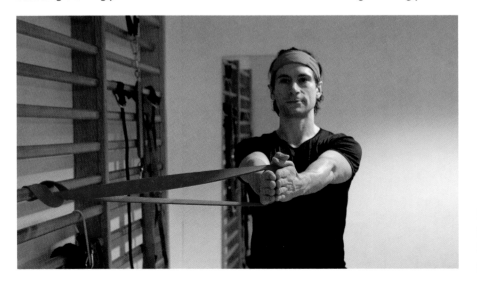

Photo 35   Palof press: thoracic stabilization in standing finishing position.

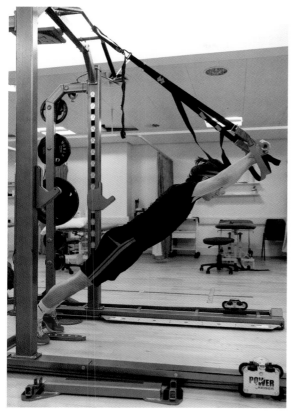

Photo 37 Suspension cable reachers, start position.

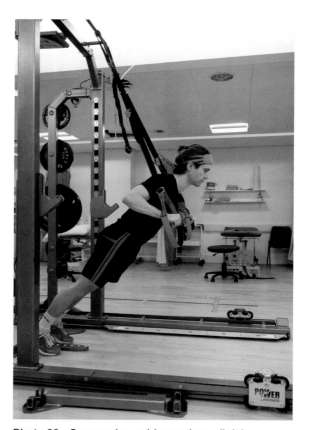

Photo 38 Suspension cable reachers, finish position.

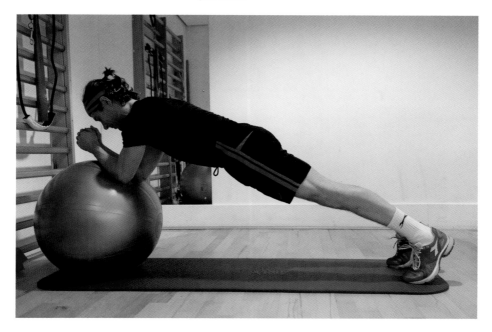

Photo 39
Sprinter's drill start position.

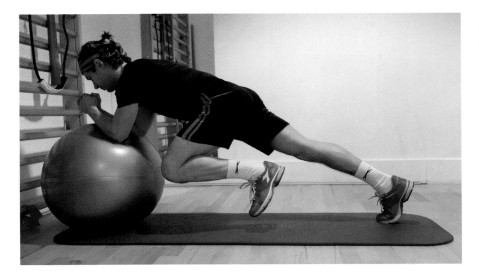

Photo 40 Sprinter's drill middle position.

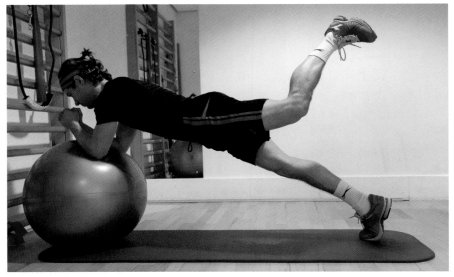

Photo 41 Sprinter's drill finishing position.

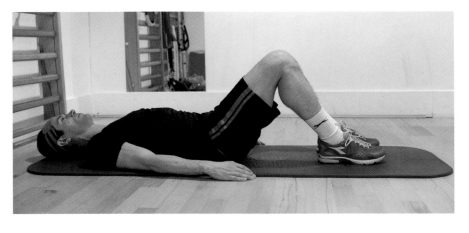

Photo 42 Supine bent knee fall-out start position.

Photo 43 Supine bent knee fall-out finish position.

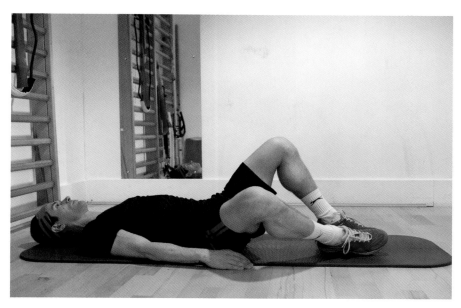

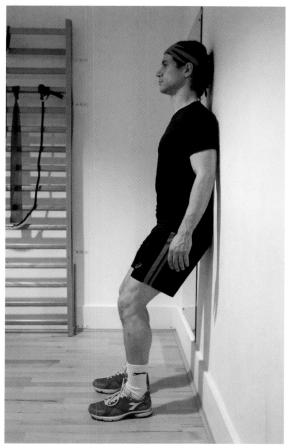

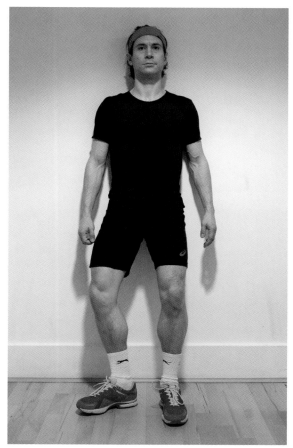

Photo 44 Standing hip dissociation start position.

Photo 45 Standing hip dissociation start position.

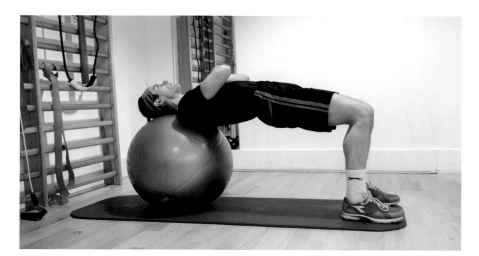

Photo 46 Swiss ball bridge starting position.

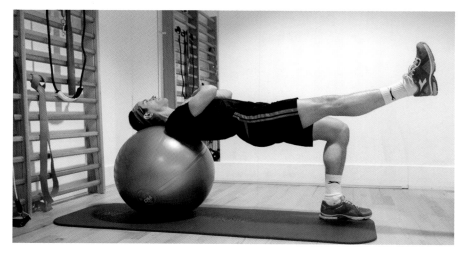

Photo 47 Swiss ball bridge middle position.

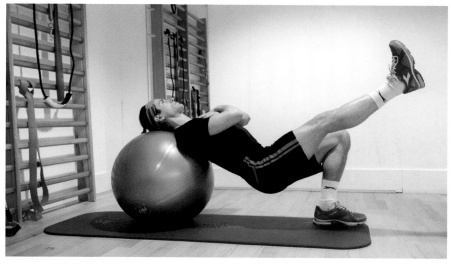

Photo 48 Swiss ball bridge finishing position.

42 and 43) and progressed into a standing position (Photos 44 and 45).

To add a loading component, the Swiss ball can be used in bridging exercises (Photos 46–48).

A Swiss ball is a useful way to provide an unstable environment to challenge the body while facilitating movement elsewhere. As dancers utilize their medial hamstrings with movements such as passé, the Swiss ball hamstring pull is an excellent exercise to stimulate a strong trunk while activating the medial hamstrings (Photos 49 and 50).

To load the lateral hamstrings more, an adjustment to the reverse Swiss ball bridge can be used (Photo 51).

The use of whole-body movement chains without exercise equipment is beneficial as it starts to lean towards the functionality required in dance. For example, the standing bird/dog with twist can be extended to include a hand-held weight (Photos 52 and 53).

Although they are more relevant to strength and endurance, loaded plate wood chops are an excel-

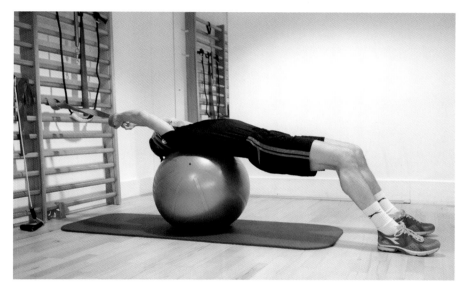

Photo 49   Swiss ball medial hamstring pull starting position.

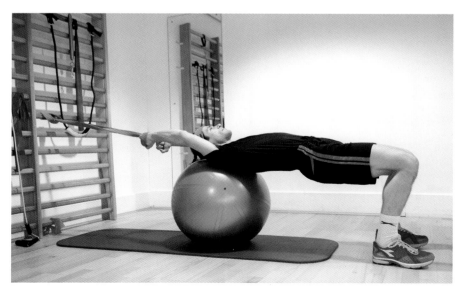

Photo 50   Swiss ball medial hamstring pull finishing position.

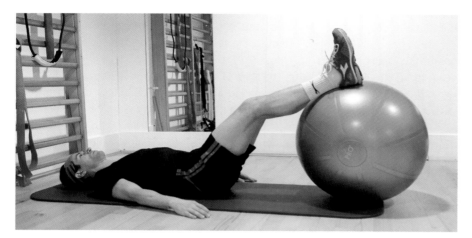

Photo 51   Reverse Swiss ball hamstring bridge start position.

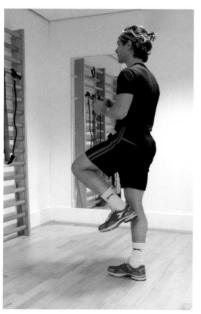

Photo 52   Standing birdman starting position.

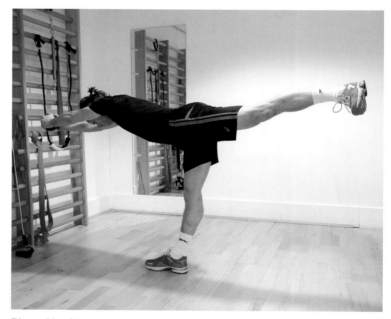

Photo 53   Standing birdman finishing position.

lent way to establish rotational stability and strength (Photos 54 and 55).

Strength

Strength is defined as the ability of a muscle or group of muscles to exert force against resistance. It is typically exerted at slower speeds (in comparison with power). The ability to sustain or maintain force (typically at sub-maximal loads) is known as strength endurance. Functional strength and strength endurance play a key role in dance performance, where dancers are frequently required to lift a partner or their own body weight, often repeatedly. Therefore, complementary strength and strength endurance training is a key component of supporting and enhancing dance performance, as well as preventing injury. Strength needs to be built on a solid foundation of optimal neuromuscular/motor

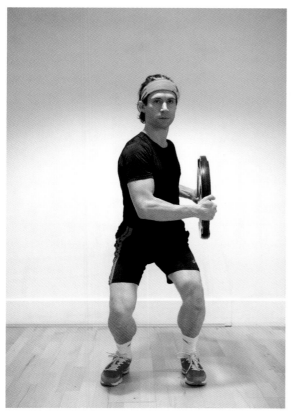

Photo 54   Standing wood chop with weight starting position.

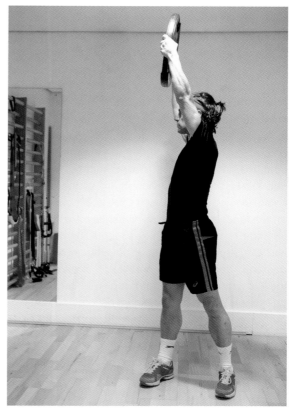

Photo 55   Standing wood chop with weight finishing position.

control stability. It can allow a dancer to hold positions and lift partners, but also provides the foundation for power work, which is needed in more ballistic movements such as jumps.

The objective for selected exercises needs to be at the forefront when designing a strength-based programme for dancers. This ensures the specificity of the programme. For some dancers, for example, the aesthetic of hypertrophy may be part of their objective for undertaking strength training. The most notable difference between strength and power training is the speed of execution in the movement. Power work is done at high velocities. Often, dance choreography asks for bursts of explosive movement, which may be repeated over a period, and these require dancers to have good power endurance. When considering the strength

and conditioning requirements for dance, it is critical to include the development of strength, power and muscle endurance.

With all exercising, warming up is important, to reduce the risk of injury and improve outputs. Strength and power training is no different. To start with, it is recommended to get the heart rate up, using static cycling or elliptical steppers perhaps. The second stage of the warm-up process involves core exercise, which can be accompanied by mobility exercises, particularly around the hips and shoulders. Finally, using a low load on the selected strength, typically up to 60 per cent of the one rep maximum (1RM) for that exercise, is a useful way to ensure the appropriate muscle groups have undergone a degree of activation and are prepared for more intense exercise.

As with all types of training, there are a multitude of variables that may be manipulated in order to achieve the desired outcome. This begins with decisions on exercise selection: for example, compound exercises such as squats or dead lifts for maximal efficiency in strength gains, as well as movement competency development, or isolation exercises to target a key muscle group, or a combination of both? The nature of the more upright dance postures, particularly in ballet, means that there may be less natural development of the posterior chain. Compound exercises such as a front squat to offer a functional carry-over with partnering (Photos 56 and 57), or Romanian dead lift (RDL) (Photos 58 and 59), are a good way of developing a dancer's posterior chain, quads and trunk strength. Once the technique and strength improve, the RDL can be progressed to a full dead lift (Photos 60 and 61), but, given the extra range in the movement, it is important that this is well controlled before being introduced.

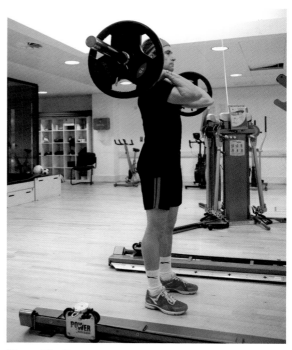

Photo 56   Front squat starting position.

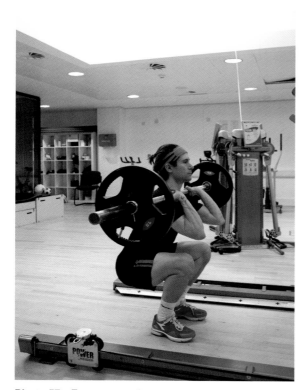

Photo 57   Front squat finishing position.

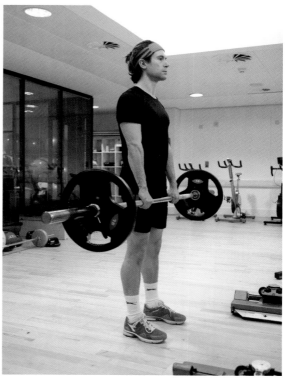

Photo 58   Romanian dead lift starting position.

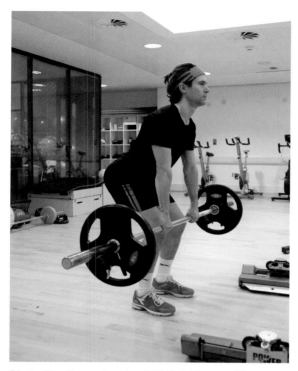

Photo 59   Romanian dead lift finishing position.

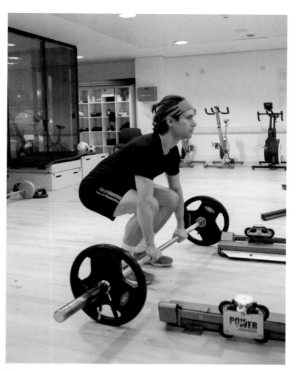

Photo 60   Dead lift starting position.

Isolation exercises can be employed where specific deficits have been identified and the programme is directed to developing a particular area, such as calf capacity (Photos 62 and 63).

Furthermore, programmes can be manipulated and adjusted using the degree of load, number of repetitions and sets, recovery times between reps and sets, tempo and speed of reps. Manipulations of the variables can assist in achieving a certain outcome. For example, adding a superset can increase the tempo of a training session by reducing recovery between sets. An unrelated set of muscles or a reciprocal muscle group can be targeted, or the same muscle group with a different exercise to create a greater loading of the target group.

Developing programmes as part of a periodized approach to a dancer's season is also important. This may mean aiming to achieve strength or power gains outside performance periods, and sustaining gains through performance periods with lower-volume programmes with higher neuromuscular emphasis.

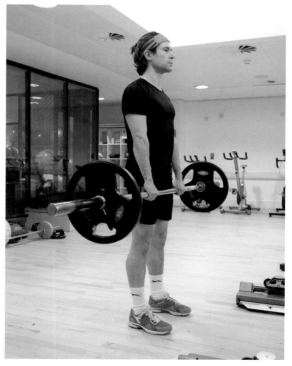

Photo 61   Dead lift finishing position.

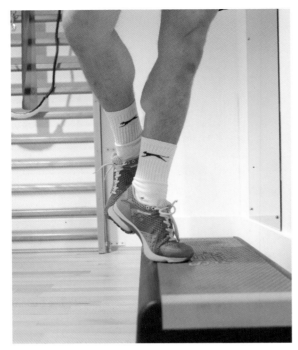

Photo 62   Calf raise in turn-out, start position.

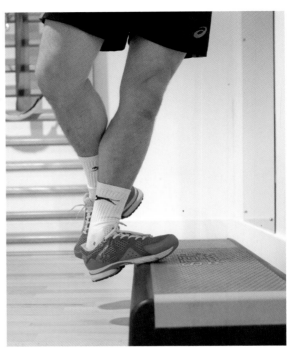

Photo 63   Calf raise in turn-out, finish position.

When prescribing exercises for strength gain, a practitioner would typically look at between 2 and 6 sets of 3 to 6 repetitions for each exercise. The load or resistance would range from 80 to 100 per cent of a one rep maximum (1RM). It is important to allow enough rest between sets in strength sessions to facilitate good recovery – up to 2 minutes if required. As dancers are often judged on how they look on stage, muscle hypertrophy may be one of their objectives. In order to achieve hypertrophy, exercises would be 3 to 4 sets of 10 repetitions. Here, the load would equate to around 80 per cent of a 1RM. If muscle endurance is the objective, then the time under load is increased. This can be achieved by undertaking 3 to 4 sets of 15 to 25 repetitions, with relatively short recovery times of around 30 seconds. Load or resistance can range from 25 to 70 per cent of the 1RM. Key to power work is the speed of movement used in the exercise. Repetitions can range from 3 to 8 reps and 3 to 5 sets, with load around 80 per cent of the 1RM.

Testing for 1RMs in untrained or unfamiliar dancers can increase the risk of injury. The National Strength and Conditioning Association in America provides a practical guide to establishing a 1RM based on repetitions at lower weights. If the dancer is able to complete 15 repetitions of a weight, this would equate to 65 per cent of their 1RM. This is further extended to 12 repetitions equating to 67 per cent of the 1RM, 6 repetitions equating to 85 per cent of the 1RM with a single repetition representing the 1RM (based on Baechle and Earle, *NSCA's Essentials of Personal Training*, 371, 2004).

In order to progress safely on to suitable strength-based load with dancers it may be appropriate to start with body-weight or even modified body-weight exercise, before moving on to greater loads. There may be occasions where the function required outweighs the available strength. The use of suspension cables can facilitate strength work where body weight is beyond loading capacity, like a pistol squat in preparation for the Trepak dance in *The Nutcracker* (Photos 64 and 65).

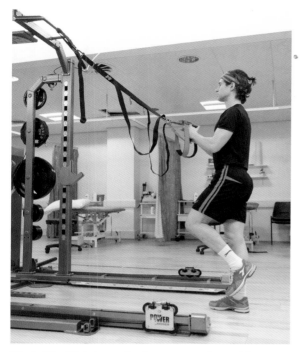

Photo 64   Pistol squat using suspension cable starting position.

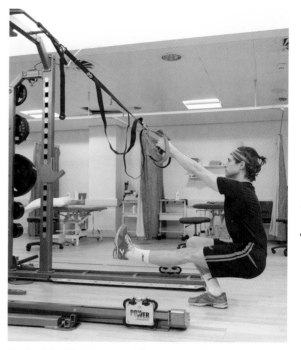

Photo 65   Pistol squat using suspension cable finishing position.

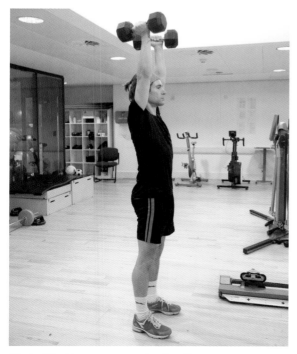

Photo 66   Hammer press in standing.

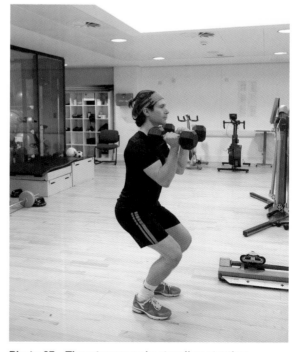

Photo 67   Thruster press in standing starting position.

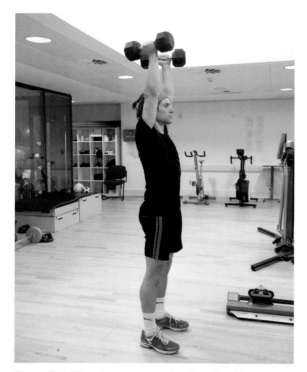

Photo 68   Thruster press in standing finishing position.

Given the functional needs in partnering and lifting, the use of hammer press (Photo 66) or thruster exercises (Photos 67 and 68) is important.

To add a more functional component to the lift, the use of water balls can help mimic the actions of a partner who, when lifted, may be required to move themselves as part of the choreography. A water ball can be made simply by filling a Swiss ball with appropriate amounts of water based on the load required (Photos 69 and 70).

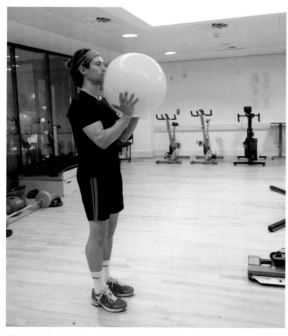

Photo 69   Water ball press and step in standing starting position.

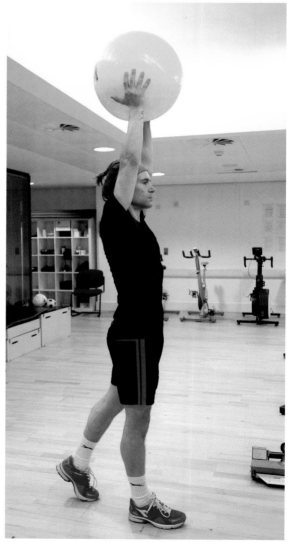

Photo 70   Water press and step in standing finishing position.

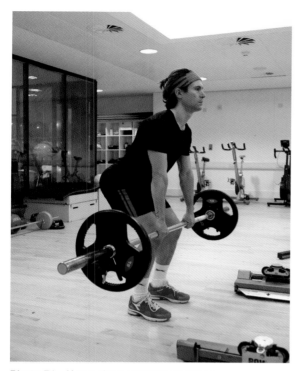

Photo 71   Hang clean starting position.

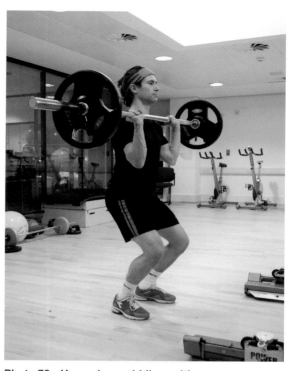

Photo 72   Hang clean middle position.

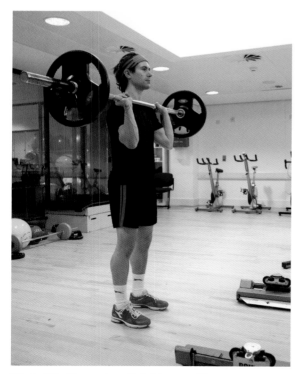

Photo 73   Hang clean finishing position.

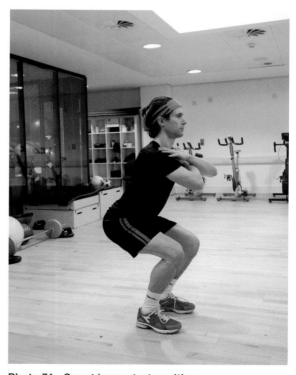

Photo 74   Squat jump start position.

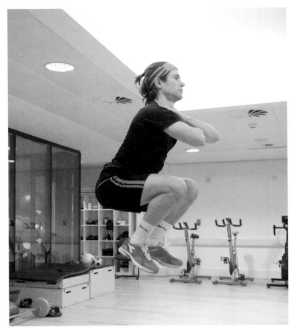

Photo 75   Squat jump finish position.

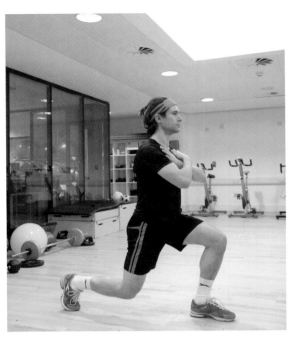

Photo 76   Split squat jump start position.

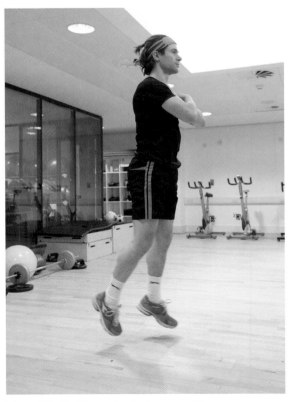

Photo 77   Split squat mid-jump position.

Power

Power development for jumping can start with compound strength work, such as squats and Romanian dead lifts. This can then be extended into a hang clean (Photos 71–73), squat jumps (Photos 74 and 75) or split squat jumps (Photos 76 and 77).

When developing power, particularly through the lower chain for jumping, ballistic drills such as pogos are useful for isolated lower-leg power development at lower loads and for warming up the system for larger jump drills (Photos 78 and 79).

When creating a more functional approach to jump training, jump boxes (Photos 80 and 81) enable the dancer to develop high explosive take-offs without the need to rely on the technical and eccentric ability to land the jump. That said, landing mechanics and eccentric muscle capacity are imperative to the whole process. They can be developed separately, allowing more concentration on the key components of the jump. The exercises can develop from simple hop and holds to jump box lands (Photos 82 and 83).

If available, doing jump drills in water to develop power endurance is an excellent option.

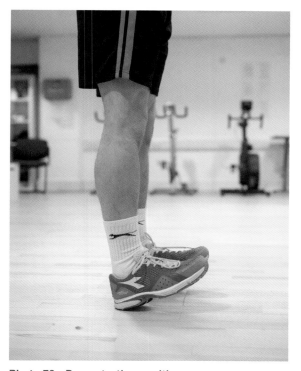

Photo 78   Pogo starting position.

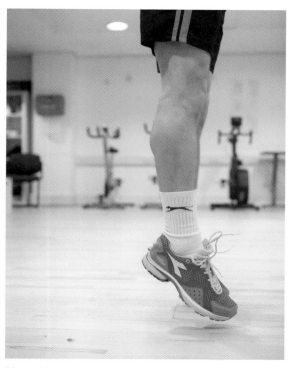

Photo 79   Pogo finishing position.

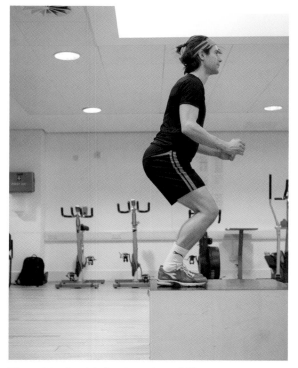

Photo 80   Double leg jump box drills.

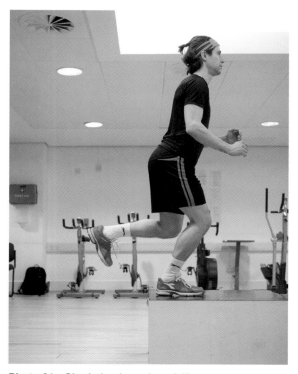

Photo 81   Single leg jump box drills.

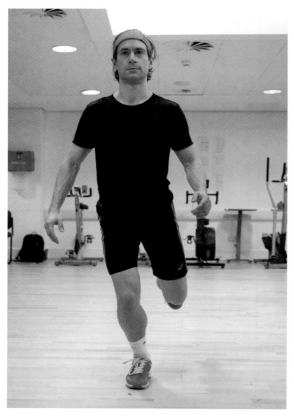

Photo 82   Hop and hold.

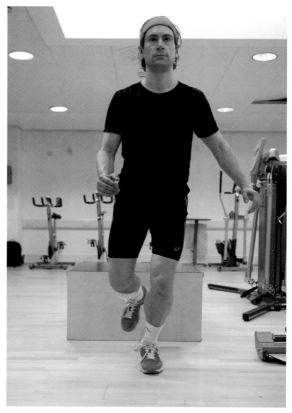

Photo 83   Jump box landing drills.

Muscle Endurance and Fitness

At rest, an average adult will be taking around 10 to 15 breaths in a minute. Each breath has a (tidal) volume of around 0.5 litres. This may vary according to body mass (and metabolic rate), as larger people require greater oxygenation. With exercise, the size of each breath is increased from 0.5 litres to 3–4 litres, while in elite endurance athletes this can be higher still, sometimes exceeding 5 litres. The maximum volume taken up and used by the body is expressed as VO2(max). In dancers, these figures have been shown by researchers to be lower than those seen in endurance athletes. Furthermore, in order to deliver the increased oxygen to the target muscle groups, an increase in cardiac output is required. Research into the fitness requirements of dance have highlighted the bursts of high-intensity exercise between longer, lower-intensity work.

Dancers therefore require both endurance, to allow them to perform lower-intensity work for prolonged periods (an average full-length ballet is around 2 hours, while a rehearsal day may be as long as 6 hours), and the fitness to perform high-intensity bouts during solo pieces or particular aspects of choreography or class. If it exceeds the lactate threshold, high-intensity exercise can have an impact on areas such as balance. Given the physiological demands, it would be sensible in training to create both a suitable aerobic base and a high lactate or anaerobic threshold.

With short-duration (lasting less than 30 seconds) high-intensity exercise and recovery times greater than around 2 minutes, there tends to be a much smaller respiratory response, as the primary energy system is ATP-PC. This may explain why, when tested, dancers do not normally demonstrate higher

VO2(max) scores, as some solo pieces and higher-intensity components in class may last less than 30 seconds, with longer recovery sessions between high-intensity bouts. However, if the exercise is sufficiently intense and long enough, as with anaerobic or muscle endurance training, an excess post-exercise oxygen consumption state (EPOC) may arise, where the oxygen debt is being corrected via an increased ventilatory state even after exercise. Managing this impact is important in dance as a dancer may be required to continue on stage after a high-intensity bout, but directed not to look flustered. A programme to support dancers may aim to build better capacity of both aerobic and anaerobic states by using interval training, which has been shown to improve aerobic capacity significantly.

Given the volume of work done by dancers in higher-impact situations, the use of non-impact modalities can provide a welcome respite for overloaded joints. This may take the form of a pool-based session where drills can be designed around the use of aqua jogging belts. The use of ergometer rowers provides an excellent way of challenging both aerobic and anaerobic capacity, as well as stimulating leg and back strength and having a positive influence on lumbar bone mineral density. The use of static bikes is another way to facilitate both aerobic and anaerobic training while providing a positive stimulus for hips and legs. With advances in technology, equipment such as the Watt Bike can offer precise programmes for dancers as well as analyse power outputs for each leg in order to monitor asymmetries.

When considering a bike to supplement fitness sessions, the dancer should be 'fitted' to it. Depending on required outcomes (power versus aerodynamic positions, for example), a number of alterations may be made to a standard bike fit, however for the purposes of supplementary fitness work, the standard fit is a good starting point:

- To determine saddle height, the subject should sit on the saddle and ensure they have a straight leg with the heel on the pedal and the pedal in the 6 o'clock position. If they are on the pedal with

the ball of the foot, they should have a 20-degree bend at the knee.
- Saddle position fore/aft can be measured by dropping a plumb line directly in front of the knee with the pedal in the 3 o'clock position – it should bisect the axis of the pedal.
- The handlebar height should allow the dancer to sit on the top bars with a small, comfortable bend at the elbows.

Bike sessions may be used to improve overall fitness and promote changes in aerobic and anaerobic capacity, but they can also help to develop power or muscle endurance. Longer sessions can be used to develop strength endurance, while high-intensity bursts can develop muscle power. The use of 'power blocks', typically high-intensity outputs at high cadence (90–110rpm) for 5 minutes followed by 5 minutes' recovery at 70–80rpm and low power outputs can be used to develop the capacity to endure the high bursts of intense jumping often seen in modern choreography. A bike session can even be made to reflect specifically the nature of a solo piece, with high-intensity sections being timed to correspond with the actual time spent at intensity in the choreography, typically from 30 seconds to 2 minutes.

Weights-based cardio sessions have also been shown to have a positive impact on both fitness and metabolic rate.

The concept of 'functional training' has become a buzz word in the fitness world. Functional is defined as 'relating to the way something works', and the purpose of functional training in dance is to provide improvements in the way in which a dancer functions. It can be very effective in improving balance, stability and movement coordination but, if strength gains are required, then isolated strength work might provide a better form of exercise. One question around functional training is whether it transfers into skill-based requirements. If the programme is designed to include aspects of the skill or movements required, this should enhance the transferable nature of the exercise. One example might be the use of pistol squats on a suspension cable system when preparing for the Trepak dance in *The Nutcracker* (*see* Photos 64 and 65). High-intensity interval sessions can include a complementary drill for the jumps and lifts seen in choreography, while also contributing to overall fitness developments.

RECOVERY

Training is the process of building resilience in the body to cope with the demands placed on it. Often, the difference between good training and an overuse injury can be effective recovery. Recovery, like training, is a multifactorial consideration. Research is often focused on investigating one recovery strategy, but the evidence to support single-modality recovery strategies, such as compression garments or ice baths, is not strong. This is further compounded by a lack of sensitive biochemical markers (typically, creatine kinase is used, which is present with muscle break-down) as a by-product of exercise to measure objectively and independent of patient-reported responses, such as delayed-onset muscle soreness (DOMS), which are susceptible to subjective influence. As a result, confidence in the implementation of some recovery strategies can be diminished. As with injury, when considering the multifactorial nature of human physiology, it stands to reason that a single-modality approach will not create changes that are statistically sufficiently significant to allow a practitioner to advocate their use without reservation. However, with an appreciation of the limitations of the research and an understanding of the physiological systems at play in exercise, it is possible to develop a multi-modal approach to recovery. This can be further individualized based on each person, the time available before the next training or performance session, and so on.

Energy Systems

Simply put, the energy source for muscle tissue is Adenosine triphosphate (ATP), which breaks down to Adenosine diphosphate (ADP) and a phosphate when releasing energy. When training intensity is sufficiently high and exceeds the recovery of the muscle energy source from ADP, a build-up of lactate occurs. The 'lactate threshold' is reached when the body can no longer reconvert ADT to ATP to keep up with energy demand and there is an exponential increase in lactate. While this is an important stimulus for various physiological changes that are seen with training, including the release of the human growth hormone that facilitates strength development, it is also important to recover well from training to reduce the risk of injury.

Recovery Strategies

An understanding of the basic energy systems allows for the planning of effective recovery strategies. In its simplest form, the reconversion of ATP requires energy and oxygen (in the presence of circulating creatine). A recovery strategy can look at barriers to this and introduce means to address and support the body's recovery. This starts with an effective warm-down. As oxygen is critical to the reconversion of ATP, having a delivery of oxygen via oxygenated blood to the target muscles is an important step. The warm-down needs to incorporate two factors. First, it needs to be set at an intensity that allows effective oxygenation. Typically, if the dancer or athlete can hold a conversation during the warm-down, they are training at a level that allows effective oxygen delivery. If using a heart rate monitor, the dancer may choose a session at 60 per cent of the HRmax. The second principle is that it needs to deliver the oxygen to the muscles that require recovery, in other words, the muscle groups used in the training session. Following a high-intensity jumping session for dance, for example, the use of a static spin bike can allow the safe delivery of oxygen to the legs without excessive joint loading or increased injury risk.

The reconversion of ADP to ATP requires oxygen but it also requires energy. The energy system can be topped up with a quick-release form of carbohydrate (shorter-chain simple carbohydrate), such as dried fruit. A carbohydrate drink or fruit snack is a useful way of providing an energy source to support the recovery of the muscle energy systems. The inclusion of longer-chain, complex carbohydrates (such as wholewheat pasta or rice) as well as protein (fish, lean chicken, and so on), is also important, to replenish energy stores and promote 'muscle repair'. The optimal timing for this is typically within an hour of the training session.

Cold submersion in ice baths and the use of contrast baths (warm and cold) have been a mainstay of recovery for many years. However, as the use of evidence-based practices increases, some high-performance institutions have reduced their reliance on this. The theoretical recovery gains from ice baths and contrast baths are via the so-called Hunting Reaction, whereby the body, in responding to the reduction in surface temperature, increases blood to the periphery (carrying oxygen to the relative region). Further speculation about its impact relates to the compressive effect of the hydrostatic pressure of being in an ice bath. A number of recent studies have suggested that the use of ice baths may have a detrimental impact on longer-term strength gain. Larger studies are needed to explore this potential more. In the absence of stronger evidence, it is important to listen to the athlete or dancer and gauge their response to any use of ice baths. If in doubt, it is probably wise to avoid this method and continue with other modalities.

Compression machines and garments have been popular for a few decades now, with advocates citing the principle of improved lymphatic drainage. The scientific evidence supporting their use is limited, but some athletes do report an improvement in delayed onset muscle soreness. Even if there is insufficient evidence supporting a biochemical change, the power of psychology to influence performance outputs should not be underestimated; similarly, it should not be dismissed in recovery. If an athlete or dancer feels that he or she recovers well using compression garments, then it would seem sensible to continue with their use.

Some sports, such as cycling, seem to use massage more than others as part of their recovery protocols. Again, there is a lack of scientific support for the implementation of this method. Advocates will point towards the impact on blood supply to target certain areas, lymphatic drainage when using effleurage, and even the psychological impact of a tactile intervention. Further to this, there appears a reasonable logical validity to 'normalizing' muscle length through stretching or myofascial releases. One prominent orthopaedic surgeon, known for his support of evidence-based medicine, advocates stretching every night before going to bed to ensure that no undue stress is placed on the muscle and joint systems while sleeping. For dancers, where range is a critical part of their daily requirements, normalizing hypertonic changes in muscle following a day's dancing or training appears to be a reasonable approach.

Combining the physiological principles and applying a multimodality approach, a typical warm-down session following a high-intensity jump-based dance session may look like this:

1. Hydration with water, recovery snack and/or drink (small portion of dried fruit and nuts, carbohydrate drink)
2. 10–15 minutes static bike (80–90rpm, 60 per cent HRmax)
3. Stretching or self-myofascial releases using roller on legs, glutes and back
4. Ice bath?
5. Compression tights/socks
6. Full meal including complex carbohydrates and protein

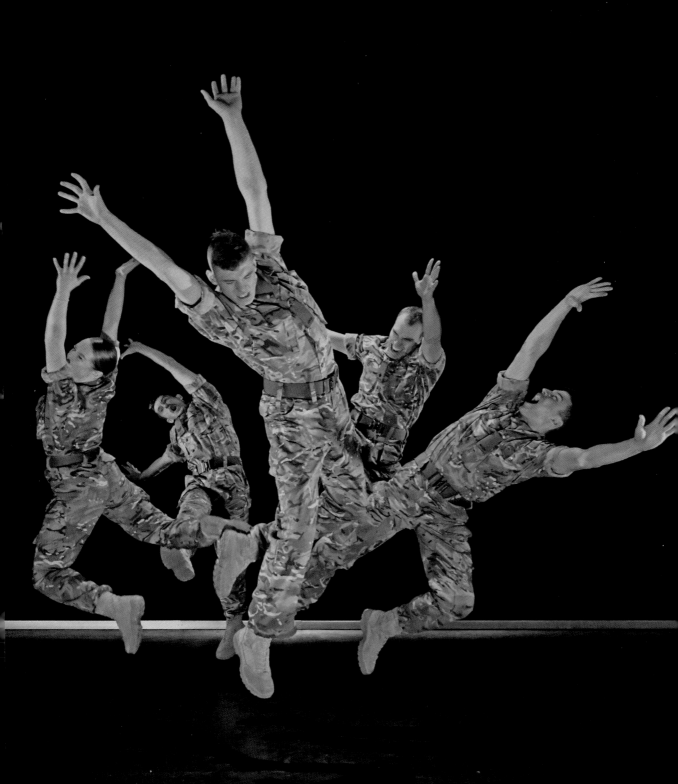

CHAPTER 5

INJURY PREVENTION, MANAGEMENT AND REHABILITATION

This chapter aims to introduce the concepts of injury prevention, with reference to the understanding gained through the injury aetiological models. It will examine the evidence and application of strategies targeting intrinsic and extrinsic risk. It will discuss injury management and highlight the risk of developing a dysfunctional injury cycle, which is often seen post-injury. It will highlight potential intervention strategies, including acute injury management, as well as a rehabilitation model from which longer-term injury rehabilitation programmes can be planned.

CONCEPTS OF INJURY PREVENTION

The aetiological models show that injury is multifactorial, starting with intrinsic risk factors that may predispose a dancer to injury, via extrinsic factors that make a dancer susceptible to injury, to an inciting event becoming the trigger (or tipping point) to injury. Injury prevention strategies need to be multifactorial too. This can be achieved through a focus on the modifiable aspects across the aetiological model, from those that make a dancer predisposed to injury (intrinsic factors), via the extrinsic factors to the inciting events.

Strategies for Intrinsic Factors

Intrinsic prevention strategies may include aspects of physical preparation such as strength, fitness and flexibility. Injury represents a point at which muscles, tendons or bones fail. It is a process along a continuum and several stages are involved on the

route to final failure. These include elastic changes, typically when tissue deforms but returns to its original state when the stressor is removed. Plastic deformation occurs when the stress to the tissue results in adaptation and changes in the original tissue. From a conditioning and preventive point of view, this is an ideal zone in which to create positive adaptive changes to build resilience in the tissue against tensile load. The final point is tissue failure when, as a result of the stress applied, tissue continuity is disrupted.

The individual failure point for the various tissues can be determined in experimental environments using a stress test. While this is useful to examine the resilience of each tissue, the nature of the stress experienced by the various tissues in the body represent a far more complex system, dependent on many factors. An injury prevention strategy needs to account for the various stressors and the points where forces may be absorbed and controlled through appropriate conditioning through the biomechanical chain.

Furthermore, the approaches used to prevent injuries can enhance performance through optimizing load transfer and force production. Typical performance models in sport reference the use of the physiological building blocks of strength, power, flexibility, and so on. Within dance there is a greater dependency on a foundation in neuromuscular training, which plays a key role in the efficiency of movement that dancers are required to demonstrate.

The use of exercise programmes as part of preventive and treatment measures for injury has been explored in the literature, with varying levels of evidence and success. The basis of exercise programmes can vary greatly, from high-threshold/resistance strength-based exercises to low-threshold proprioception-based ones. There is an increased focus today on the core stability muscles and their role in preventing injuries. Core stability has been defined as 'the ability of the lumbo-pelvic hip complex to prevent buckling and to return to equilibrium after perturbation'. The authors go on to say that 'although static elements (bone and soft tissue) contribute to some degree, core stability is predominantly maintained by the dynamic function of muscular elements', and that there is 'a clear relationship between trunk muscle activity and lower extremity movement'. What this definition provides is a description of how core stability works and the role it plays in providing support to a key body region within athletic movement. Mottram and Comerford expand on the term 'core stability' with the more comprehensive term of 'motor control stability', which is defined as 'central nervous system modulation of efficient integration and low threshold recruitment of local and global muscles systems'. A component of this may arise from neuromuscular control, which is defined as 'the unconscious efferent response to an afferent signal regarding dynamic joint stability'. The delineation of core stability to motor control stability and neuromuscular control allows the inclusion of body regions other than the lumbar pelvic region to be incorporated in the principle providing stability for athletic performance.

Although the definitions are sometimes used interchangeably, the use of motor control stability, neuromuscular control and core stability has been explored and has been suggested to be effective in the prevention of injuries and in enhancing performance. Mottram and Comerford explain the differences between motor control stability and strengthening, and indicate that strength training relates to 'high-load or high-speed training of symmetrical limb loading and asymmetrical trunk loading'. While there is evidence of the benefits of both systems, motor control stability can achieve local or global stability with stimulation of afferent spindle input affecting tonic muscle output via central nervous system process under a low load. This can provide safer and potentially quicker protection against injury, with a lower risk of concomitant injury through the use of higher resistance loads, or the time to adaptation needed for hypertrophic/strength changes with traditional strength training. Further to this, evidence has indicated that, while high-threshold training as used in traditional strength training does not appear to rectify motor control dysfunction, these can be corrected through the application of low-threshold training, such as motor control stability.

Neuromuscular training has been described as a multi-interventional programme that includes combinations of balance, core stability, strength, plyometric, agility and sport-specific exercises. It may be applied as a rehabilitation programme to restore neuromuscular control after joint injury or as a prehabilitation programme, whereby the initiation of neuromuscular exercises after joint trauma may restore function and prevent degenerative changes later. Various systematic reviews, including one Cochrane Database Systematic Review, have demonstrated the positive value of neuromuscular training in performance enhancement, sports injury prevention, injury prevention in the lumbar region, lower limb injuries, anterior cruciate ligaments (ACL) (in female athletes), and ankle instability and ankle sprain prevention.

The evidence is still limited by small sample sizes, methodological flaws, less than optimal measures used, heterogeneity of population groups and inconsistencies. Furthermore, none of the studies was based on a dancing population. Despite these limitations, however, an exercise programme that does not require equipment would be beneficial for a dance company that is touring nationally or internationally. Moreover, an exercise programme that may be effective in reducing both non-contact and overuse injuries – both injury types that are particularly noted in dance – provides a compelling case for its inclusion in an injury prevention strategy.

Implementing an effective injury prevention programme in dance is challenging. The pre-season component of the year lasts only two weeks in some professional companies, during which the dancers need to prepare for the rigours of 6 hours of rehearsals a day on top of 1½ hours of class. There is not enough time to provide sufficient strength gains through traditional strength training. Incorporating high-load training of the type used in traditional strength training during this period may also increase the risk of concomitant injury. The added challenge for many dancers is how to prepare for the athletic requirements of the season without great hypertrophic muscle gains (which have been noted with prolonged strength training), so that they can conform to the aesthetic requirements of traditional classical ballet.

There are similar challenges involved in providing injury prevention within the working season, including the extreme time constraints on dancers when it comes to complementary conditioning. Generally, the exposure time for dance-related activities is far greater than that seen in other professional sporting disciplines. As a result, an intervention that incorporates low-threshold training (to provide stability to local and global stability muscles), with a safe level of training (evident in neuromuscular training), would be advantageous.

Strategies for Extrinsic Factors

Often, extrinsic risk factors are considered to be non-modifiable. While changes to extrinsic factors may be more challenging, their potential impact on injury is well documented and needs serious consideration. Unlike many sports, the role of teammates and opposition players is less relevant within this aspect of the aetiological model. However, collisions do take place and ensuring that dancers are adequately prepared for the performance will reduce the risk of injury. Injury reduction strategies should also be targeted at those dancers involved with partnering. Partnering is a dynamic process in which both dancers require good technique, control and strength.

Susceptibility to risk may also arise from costumes, footwear and props. The key objective of costumes in dance is to enhance the story-telling as opposed to enhancing performance, which is the case in sport. It is important for the healthcare practitioner to explore and discuss any costume challenges in upcoming roles. For example, the use of a weighted vest in preparation for a role that requires a heavy coat to be worn can be an important part of injury prevention. Ensuring that the costumes allow the required movement for the choreography, including lifting and jumping, can also reduce the risk of injury.

Footwear is another challenging area in dance. Of course, the dancer needs to develop the appropriate strength and control to perform choreography en pointe, but the risk of injury will be significantly increased if the pointe shoes are not correctly sized. Insufficient space in the toe box may cause an increased risk of a Morton's neuroma, while a failure to support the midfoot adequately will increase load through the tibialis posterior and the navicular.

Props, including swords and other weapons, are often used in dance. Ensuring adequate preparation and technical proficiency in their use is an important part of an injury prevention strategy.

The surfaces on which dancers perform can vary considerably. The challenges posed by this aspect of performance relate to two key areas: the basic construction and the covering surface. In terms of basic structure, some venues in the UK have a stage with a 'rake', where the stage is tilted around 4 degrees towards the audience, to give them a better view of the performance. This tilt changes the biomechanics for the performing artists. An injury prevention strategy might involve preparation work on a slope to ensure dancers become familiar with the alteration in forces that they will experience.

The second issue in construction relates to the energy return and force-reduction properties of the floor. The ideal force reduction for dance floors is recommended to be 60 per cent, but dancers may find themselves rehearsing in community halls or non-dance studios that do not offer those ideal properties. Dancers in larger companies may rehearse in custom-built studios that do comply with the recommendations, but the challenge to them arises when performing in multi-use theatres that were constructed to house different shows as well as heavy scenery. Furthermore, the construction beneath the sprung surface may result in inconsistencies in the floor. In some areas, there may be good force-reduction properties, while in others, particularly where the basic construction beams cross, there may be a reduction in quality. Such inconsistencies in the surface can lead to an increase in injuries. Although this may be outside the remit of many healthcare practitioners, they may be well placed to advise companies on the commissioning of the construction of a touring floor that can provide consistency with a dance-specific studio, as well as adhering to the ideal force-reduction properties needed for performances.

Additional consideration needs to be given to the surface covering the floor, which is often a lino-based product. The potential for inconsistency with the rehearsal studio surface is significant. Injury prevention strategies here may include the use of 'functional proprioception' work.

Strategies for Inciting Events

Strategies to reduce risk at the inciting event can involve both intrinsic and extrinsic factors. Involving intrinsic factors may mean improving joint kinematics during jumping and landing. Dancers will generally demonstrate higher skill levels than many sportsmen or women in this activity, but additional training of their jump and in particular landing mechanics can reduce injuries. The use of jump boxes is ideal as it allows the two major components of the jump – take-off and land – to be isolated and developed. With the 'jump up' activity, the focus can be on developing the power required for jumping. This will entail using the higher jump box stack, encouraging the participant to use and develop the explosive component in the jump without the consequential technical requirement needed for the land from a greater height. With 'jump down', the drills should focus on landing mechanics, starting initially from a lower box and progressing to a box of a simi-

lar height to the 'jump up' capacity. Typically, these drills can be progressed from double-leg take-off to double-leg land, to single-leg take-off to double-leg land, and finally single-leg take-off to single-leg land.

Once the physical resilience of the jump has been enhanced through isolated and concentrated training, it needs to be taken back into the studio for technical integration. Technical input from dance staff should be utilized to assess and give direction on omissions that may be associated with increased risk, such as a dancer failing to get the heels down during jump landing. Skill delivery is a key parameter in increased risk within the 'inciting event' component of the injury model. Due to the high level of skill demonstrated by most dancers, it may be necessary for technical or dance staff to propose changes to reduce the risk of injury.

The inciting events risk is also related to training and performance timetabling. It is quite likely that little can be done to influence the volume and timing of performance periods for many dancers. However, examining the training load may enable the practitioner to establish whether insufficient chronic training load may have played a part in this being a risk when the dancer experiences an increase in acute training due to an upcoming dance performance period. By recording chronic training load, even as an exponent of exposure (both dance-related and non-dance-related training) and intensity, the healthcare professional can begin to explore the role of manipulating chronic training load to reduce the risk of injury due to training or performance schedules.

INJURY MANAGEMENT OF A DANCER

When managing injury in a dancer, it is important to establish a working diagnosis with a clear understanding of the origin of symptoms. The site of pain or even structural disruption may not be representative of the whole picture, and an assessment of load through the entire biomechanical chain is critical to identifying potential causation. The impact of many factors can create a dysfunctional biomechani-

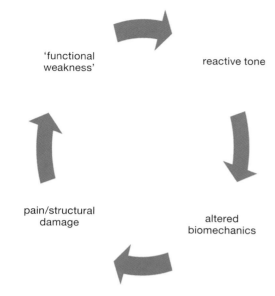

Fig. 2 Dysfunctional biomechanical cycle.

'functional weakness'

reactive tone

pain/structural damage

altered biomechanics

cal chain (Fig. 2), which can result in a confounding presentation relating to 'cause and effect' in the accurate diagnosis of injuries. It is important therefore to employ a longitudinal and reactive assessment. This entails a constant re-evaluation of the kinetic system, to ensure all contributing factors within cause and effect are monitored as the injury progresses through the various stages, from acute to end.

If the injury is assessed as being structural in origin, a further evaluation of the origin of symptoms as potentially chemical (inflammatory) or mechanical (tissue stressing through loading), or both, will assist in the management process and rehabilitation design. In traumatic injuries, there may be an expectation of a chemical origin due to tissue trauma following an inciting event. In overuse injuries, the influence of biomechanical loading in the development of symptoms is most likely, with a combined presentation of chemical and mechanical origin. Dancers present with a significant prevalence of overuse injuries. This requires the examining clinician to undertake a thorough biomechanical assessment, to establish origin and causation.

Acute Injury Management

The evolution of RICE (Rest, Ice, Compression, Elevation) to POLICE (Protect, Optimal Loading, Ice, Compression, Elevation) in acute injury represents a growing understanding of the role of optimal loading as opposed to rest. Optimal loading needs to be balanced against and comes after protection as an intervention. Protection is a critical part of acute injury management. This may involve, for example, the use of a pneumatic walker boot in the initial 24 hours of an acute ankle sprain. As well as protecting the damaged structures, it is important to support those that are now under risk due to the reduced structural integrity of the injured area. Furthermore, it is vital to create an optimal environment for healing. As always, this needs to be balanced against the impact on chronic training load, given the potential reduction in training during the early stages of rehabilitation. A period of immobilization may negatively impact on chronic training load. However, that period of immobilization may speed up a return to training, through the adequate support of damaged structures, and may therefore have a positive impact on the quality of training undertaken down the line. Communicating the concept of early injury management that includes optimal loading can allay any fears the dancer may have around the loss of training time.

Compression can be achieved using a number of items, ranging from simple compression bandages to the commercially available units, which allow greater degrees of pressure with the potential additional of cooling. Compression, like elevation, can assist in lymphatic drainage, particularly during a period where mobility and function may be comprised and the impact of muscle action on lymphatic drainage reduced.

Chronic Injury Management

As with acute injury, the management in a chronic case is dependent on the injury presentation. A dysfunctional biomechanical cycle and the biomechanics of tissue injury can result in a confounding presentation as to which is cause and which is effect when it comes to symptoms and even tissue damage (*see* Fig. 17). Chronic injury management also needs to consider the impact of detraining as part of the overall presentation. A dancer with diminished strength or power may experience loading of a resolving injured area and report very similar symptoms, but the failure to control the loading will be the cause of the pain rather than pathology.

REHABILITATION OF A DANCER

The rehabilitation of any athlete is a multifactorial process, involving numerous considerations, including the nature and severity of the injury, predisposing factors, time in season and career, and previous injury, among other factors. Applying dance specificity to traditional aetiological models allows the practitioner to formulate a strategy for the rehabilitation process that accounts for some areas that are not necessarily seen in other sporting populations. These include the challenges that have already been discussed, such as intrinsic factors (hypermobility, body composition, and so on), extrinsic factors (raked stages, pointe shoes, costumes), and inciting events (choreography, genre/style of dance or repertoire). Using all these, along with a detailed history and clinical examination, the healthcare professional can formulate ideas around the injury diagnosis and possible causative factors, as well as the functional outcomes required by the athlete or dancer for a safe return, including reducing the risk of recurrence.

The construction of injury management programmes with rehabilitation timelines needs to take into account both biological timelines (in other words, the healing time of any tissues damaged) and physiological timelines, where the physiological demands of the functional requirements (and the time required to achieve the necessary conditioning to allow this) are included in the overall programme timeline.

Exit criteria for the progression through the various levels of rehabilitation are an important part of the rehabilitation process. Setting clear goals for patients to work towards, with suitably appropriate exit criteria or achievement criteria to which they can progress, the next incremental level of loading and rehabilitation ensures that patients progress at the correct times and can reduce the risk of delayed rehabilitation due to exacerbation or subsequent injury.

A planning document to demonstrate clear but flexible progression is an important tool. Using a weekly timeline, the various stages in the biological and functional progression plan can be plotted. The initial stage starts (according to the POLICE protocol) with a period of Protection/Optimal Loading. This may be for an initial period of two weeks, post-surgery, while protecting wound sites and surgical repairs, and so on. This is a clinical rehabilitation period with close monitoring, particularly in surgical patients.

This stage is followed by a period of load accumulation. In this phase there is the initiation of load, preparing the rehabilitating dancer to train suitably for what they will be required to do. Facilitation of normal movement patterns are key in this phase. This includes obtaining the required range of movement, as the injury allows, as well as competency of more compound movements. Furthermore, it plays a role, through functional loading, in developing the orientation of fibres in healing tissue. This stage may last only a couple of weeks, depending on the pathology and procedures undertaken.

The load accumulation stage is followed by a dance-specific strength and movement phase. This is the 'train-to-train' phase and incorporates the progression of movement competency, and the development of strength and power, with further extension to include strength and power endurance. As part of the power development, it also incorporates jump competency development. As this phase is focused on developing changes in physiological parameters, it is critical to allow enough time for the changes to take place. Typically, it may require 6 weeks.

This phase is followed by the functional integration phase, the 'train-to-perform' phase. This is characterized by a focus on dance-specific rehabilitation, including a return to studio-based work in the form of technical coaching and class participation.

Work undertaken during the dance-specific strength and movement phase, which may have included pool-based barre work, for example, is part of the development of skill and capacity that will allow the dancer to proceed to studio-based technical work within the Functional Integration phase. This phase is used to consolidate jump and pointe work as well as reinforce any technical adjustments made through the coaching sessions.

The appropriate level of loading based on the stage of the injury can be established by an evaluation of what the limiting factor is at that time. In other words, what is stopping the patient from undertaking all that they would normally do? In the case of an acute injury, it may be pain and structural damage that determines the degree of impairment. In overuse or chronic injuries, it may be an underlying strength or power deficit or a limited functional capacity due to lack of appropriate training.

HYBRID INTERVENTION MODEL

The Hybrid Intervention Model (HIM) is a theoretical model designed to allow clinicians to plan the strategies that they wish to employ through the injury and rehabilitation process.

The nature of the intervention for dancers needs to conform to three main factors. The primary factor is functional outcomes. This means that the intervention, although it is not always required to be dance-specific, does need to reduce injuries within dance-related activities. Second, the intervention needs to be achievable, within the time restraints imposed on the dancer and within the limits of the injury itself. This takes into account pre-season and in-season scheduling, where time allocation for complementary training is extremely limited. Third, the intervention needs to respect the aesthetic requirements of dance, where the body shape that results from hypertrophic change due to strength training could be considered unacceptable.

A neuromuscular training-based intervention programme will enable the dancer to achieve the required functional outcomes. Several systematic reviews have demonstrated the benefits of neuromuscular training in performance enhancement and injury prevention. Research has suggested that both strength and fitness levels in dancers are poor in comparison with other elite level sports participants. Yet the performance output of these dancers suggests that there is another means by which they are able to perform such athletic feats over such an extended period of time. Questions may be raised over the validity of some traditional strength and fitness-based tests in terms of dance, but it has been suggested that the performance outputs in dance, in the absence of higher levels of strength or fitness, are due a very high level of skill. This level of skill may allow athletic movements to be performed with the greatest degree of efficiency, thereby reducing the need for higher levels of strength or fitness.

One major component of the neuromuscular training approach is the activation of the correct muscles. This is to provide a stabilizing of the joints, which reduces the need for compensatory and/or over-activation of other muscle groups. This over- or incorrect activation of muscle groups for the purpose of providing joint stability leads to poor efficiency of energy and harnessing of muscle power. As dancers have been perceived as naturally demonstrating enhanced efficiency, implementing a training programme that complements their natural training would seem to provide the best opportunity to achieve the required outcome. It is felt that correct motor control function, allowing the high level of skill, is critical to the normal resilience of dancers to injury. As such, an intervention where support for the use of low-threshold training, such as motor control stability/neuromuscular control in the correction of motor control dysfunction, has been demonstrated, would enable the achievement of the primary objective of improved functional outcome of reduced dance-related injuries.

One component of motor control stability/ neuromuscular control arises from the role of afferent nerves. Mandelbaum et al. indicated that the afferent signals have two distinctive roles: feedback and feed-forward mechanisms. Feed-forward mechanisms are a result of a preparatory activation of muscle, as opposed to the slower, more reflexive feedback mechanism elicited through the afferent input of force to joint. The feed-forward aspect of neuromuscular control is a key component that can be utilized for injury prevention strategies. The preparatory aspect of feed-forward neuromuscular control seems to allow changes in resilience to injury to be achieved in a shorter time period than the adaptive muscle changes that result from a strength-based exercise intervention approach. It also eliminates the potential of unwanted hypertrophic muscle changes that could adversely affect the aesthetic requirements of the individual dancers. A motor control stability/neuromuscular control approach to the intervention strategy achieves the correct sequencing of exercise types. In this process, the establishment of local and global stabilization prior to the engagement of any higher-threshold intervention not only allows a more effective gain to be made from the progression of exercises, due to the creation of a suitable 'platform' on which functional and higher-threshold exercises may be based, but also reduces the risk of concomitant injury that might occur when applying a higher-threshold loading of the body without establishing that stabilization.

The HIM was developed through observation of key performance attributes from elite sport and elite dance and based on the principles of neuromuscular training. It was important to ensure that the same model could be applied to the design of a conditioning programme for dancers with an injury as well as for dancers for whom an injury risk was identi-fied. The model incorporates the skill and efficiency of movement observed in elite dancers with the strength and fitness identified in elite sports participants. The 'hybrid' looks to combine movement efficiency with strength training within the programme.

The hybrid model uses three points of consideration for each programme (Fig. 3):

1. the injury (if there is an injury present) or deficit (as identified through the audit and screening processes);
2. the cause (of the injury or deficit); and
3. the final objective or outcome being sought as a result of undertaking the programme.

All three factors need to be considered in the construction of an intervention programme, but the model also seeks to identify which of the three is the key 'limiting factor' for the current stage of the injury/deficit (for example, the acute/early stage, the sub-acute/mid stage, or the chronic/late stage). This then influences the relative ratios of the three factors that are combined to form each programme or session, namely neuromuscular facilitation, isolated segmental deficit training and functional integration. In the early stage of an injury or an identified deficit, the key limiting factor may be the injury or the deficit itself. At this stage, the cause and the end-stage objective carry less weight. The resulting programme then focuses on neuromuscular facilitation as its largest component, with smaller components addressing the segmental deficit and functional integration.

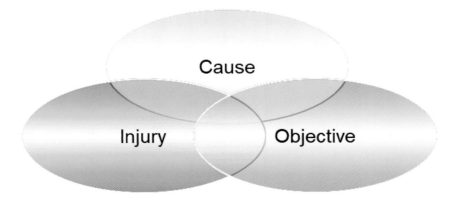

Fig. 3 **Three points of consideration in musculoskeletal injury.**

The development of correct neuromuscular control and movement efficiency patterns is required to provide a safe foundation to load an injured or deficient region, without risk of injury or compensatory movement or muscular patterns. The segmental deficit component identifies the muscle group/s within the movement chain that influence the overall functioning, but are deficient, and looks to improve their isolated function. It is hypothesized that, in the presence of a segmental deficit, movement can be achieved with similar functional outcomes, but with degrees of compensatory movements that may entail potential risk of injury or diminished performance.

The last component of the conditioning programme incorporates 'functional integration'. This uses the establishment of improved neuromuscular firing patterns and isolated strengthening and immediately challenges these in functional positions. In the early stages these may be in unloaded postures that mimic or replicate functional activities like running or jumping.

As the individual progresses through the training periods, the shift in the limiting factors is reflected in the construction of the conditioning programme. In the mid stage of the training period, the limiting factor may no longer be the injury/deficit, and the cause begins to carry more weight. The conditioning programme will see a slightly smaller component addressing the neuromuscular firing patterns, and a more significant emphasis on any segmental deficit, along with a slightly greater shift towards functional integration.

At the end stage, the injury/deficit as well as the cause should be less influential, and the main limiting factor will come from the proposed outcome or objective. For a dancer, this objective may be a return to full performance on stage. At this stage, the conditioning programme sees less emphasis on the neuromuscular and segmental deficit components and more emphasis on the functional integration. Despite the shift towards the functional integration, the programme design still allows for on-going work within the neuromuscular and segmental deficit aspects. This is done to ensure the on-going efficiency of the movement patterns alongside the strength and function work. This hybrid approach is considered key to improving performance outcomes and reducing (re)injury risk. Notable throughout the conditioning programme but emphasized in the third phase is the need to perform exercises with efficiency and no compensatory movements.

The progression through the programme relies on changes/improvements to the pre-test determinant. The result of the Mens test and the role of the sacroiliac joint can be fundamental to a lumbo-pelvic to lower-leg rehabilitation programme. The presence of a positive Mens test would normally form the foundation for the first phase and the development of the motor control/firing patterns of the muscles that provide stability to the sacroiliac joint. Gluteus maximus and piriformis muscles have been advocated as playing a key role in improving force closure of the sacroiliac joint and in the subsequent improvement in stability, and can be used to facilitate this action. In order to achieve progression to the next exercises, dancers should be instructed to repeat the Mens test and only to proceed if the test has improved – if, for example, the leg feels lighter or equal. The exercises in the segmental deficit portion of the programme are designed to add support for the muscle groups needed to maintain sacroiliac

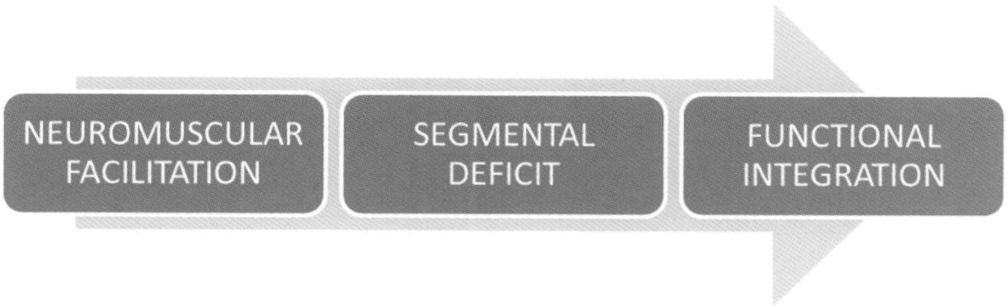

Fig. 4   Individual components making up the Hybrid Intervention Model programme.

NEUROMUSCULAR FACILITATION

SEGMENTAL DEFICIT

FUNCTIONAL INTEGRATION

joint stability as well as address the concurrent deficiencies noted, while the final portion of the programme looks to challenge those key areas in a functional biomechanical posture.

The hybrid model proposes the implementation of three strands to each programme delivered: neuromuscular foundation training, strength/power (including strength or power endurance), and functional integration (Fig. 4). The keys to the implementation of the model are the sequence (neuromuscular followed by strength followed by functional integration), and the relative ratios of the different components at each stage of the injury episode. The relative ratios are influenced by the clinician's assessment of the current limiting factor.

Hybrid Intervention Model: Early Stage

In the early stage of an acute injury the likely limiting factor, and as such focus of the management programme, is the injury itself and any associated pain. One notable result of pain in acute injury is the impact on muscle inhibition. Within the HIM, neuromuscular facilitation represents the most significant component of the rehabilitation programme, to restore and support muscle activa-

tion during this key time. Neuromuscular exercise is typically well tolerated in the presence of pain and therefore fits well in the early stages (Fig. 5).

Hybrid Intervention Model: Mid Stage

As a patient progresses through the injury stages, the next limiting factor and management focus may be the cause of the injury. At the mid stage, the identification and addressing of any potential strength or power deficits may make up the largest proportion of the programme design (Fig. 6).

At this stage, the programme will still begin with muscle activation drills, with some functional activation drills at the end of the session. The promotion of strength (or power) gains relies on a principle of overload – creating a load great enough to challenge the targeted structures to stimulate adaptation and change. Conventional understanding is that stimulating change in muscle tissue to promote increases in strength requires a repetition of load around 60–80 per cent of the one rep max (1RM), where the 1RM is the greatest load the patient could lift once. If the load is too great in the presence of an injury at this stage of the rehabilitation process, there may be an increased risk of exacerbation or more pain.

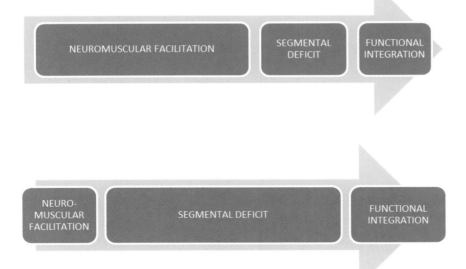

Fig. 5   Early-stage Hybrid Intervention Model ratios.

Fig. 6   Mid-stage Hybrid Intervention Model ratios.

BLOOD FLOW RESTRICTION TRAINING

One alternative option that can provide a suitable physiological stimulus to promote changes in muscle tissue but at a much lower load (20 per cent of the 1RM) is blood flow restriction training (BFRT). BFRT is the process of using a device such as a blood pressure cuff to reduce the amount of oxygenation to the target muscle group, creating a relative hypoxic state for the muscle energy systems. The reduced oxygenation during low-load training stimulates the release of the human growth hormone, a key mediator in the strength development process.

The risk associated with BFRT has been equated to that of resistance training, but it is important to carry out an additional screening process. Patients with a history of blood-clotting disorders, deep vein thrombosis or pulmonary embolus, vascular or nerve trauma or haemorrhagic stroke would be considered to be at high risk in using BFRT. They may be excluded from this type of training, or have to employ means to mitigate the risk, including reduced training time under cuff pressure, lower cuff pressure, or using intermittent rather than constant pressure. Patients with a history of smoking or use of the contraceptive pill, and those who have recently taken a long-haul flight may be at increased risk of a DVT. They would be considered a medium risk, and should also consider reducing training time under cuff pressure, lowering cuff pressure, or using intermittent rather than constant pressure.

A standardized questionnaire should be used to screen all patients prior to any such training, to determine the appropriateness of BFRT. Patients must also be made aware of the possible side effects, which range from delayed onset muscle soreness, which is typical, to rhabdomyolysis, which the literature suggests is rare.

As the understanding of BFRT increases, prescription around sets and repetitions may become more specific. Current guidelines suggest that time spent under restrictive blood flow should be limited to around 15 minutes. A typical programme might include one set of 30 repetitions, followed by three sets of 15 repetitions of each exercise directed at the target muscle group, up to a total of 15 minutes. One example, for a lower-limb programme post an anterior cruciate ligament (ACL) reconstruction, with the objective of working on leg strength, may include 1 x 30 squats, 3 x 15 squats, 1 x 30 Romanian dead lifts (RDLs), 3 x 15 RDLs, and so on.

Hybrid Intervention Model: End Stage

In the final stages of a rehabilitation programme, the focus and management shift towards the functional requirements of the athlete or dancer for their safe return to performance or competition. A shorter muscle activation and strength-based programme will be followed by an extended functionally driven component (Fig. 7).

A further consideration in the rehabilitation of dancers is the need to optimize loading as part of their preparation and resilience training. This is a key part of the functional integration compo-

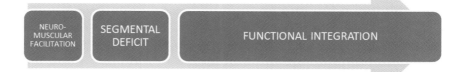

Fig. 7   End-stage Hybrid Intervention Model ratios.

nent of the HIM. It encompasses both the creation of suitable chronic load through the rehabilitation programme, to build resilience for the inevitable spikes in acute workload that are seen in dance and especially in performance. This includes an appreciation of the impact of career loading – the loading of previous seasons, alongside chronic training load from the last four weeks. Research suggests that younger athletes may be at an increased risk of injury through a lack of suitable chronic training load, while older athletes may be more at risk due to either excessive accumulative chronic loading or previous injury affecting training load. Research also suggests that spikes in acute workload may result in increased bone stress injury. This may be particularly notable in younger dancers, who do not yet possess the chronic workload to support against these spikes. On the other hand, accumulative excessive chronic workload may result in increased risk of pathological changes to joint surfaces; this is an area that may be more relevant to dancers who are further into their career. All these factors need to be taken into account when designing rehabilitation programmes for dancers, alongside the criteria for return to dance.

RETURN TO DANCE CRITERIA

It is well understood that previous injury is one of the biggest risks to re-injury and subsequent injury. A return to the previous level of participation is usually seen as a successful outcome for rehabilitation.

When determining the return to play criteria for a sportsperson, it is usually straightforward to identify the physical state that is required for full return, as there is a relative degree of consistency in the nature of competition (although it can be affected by the opposition). In dance, the nature of the choreography and the specific roles can vary considerably. Due to the huge variation in the physiological demands of the different choreographies, a decision for a dancer to return to performance requires a full understanding of the demands of the role to which he or she will be returning. If a graded return is being considered (for example, if

the role does not require full physical capacity), it is important to clarify that the return to performance is caveated around completion of the rehabilitation process before full dance participation can be considered.

As in sports, decisions around any return need to involve a team made up of the dancer, the artistic staff, and the clinical and conditioning staff. Artistic staff may be able to clarify the likely physical demands on the dancer in upcoming rehearsal and performance roles, but it is also important to understand the dancer's perspective. There must be an awareness of their view on their contracts, career development and performance pressure.

Limb Symmetry Testing

From a clinical perspective, an adaptation of a commonly used sports model may guide the decision process. In the absence of pre-season baseline data, the use of limb symmetry index testing can provide a useful reference point for injuries to lower and upper limbs. A limb symmetry index of within 25 per cent gives some suggestion of a reduced risk of injury based on the literature from ACL rehabilitation and RTP protocols; a deficit of 10 per cent or under of the unaffected side gives stronger confidence that there will be no performance deficit. The content of the tests can be adjusted to suit other pathologies, but may include the following for the lower limb:

- **Normal movement:** functional movement testing to assess movement competency and neuromuscular control.
- **Range of movement (ROM):** hip ROM (particularly internal rotation as an exponent of how the external rotators of the hip are coping). Knee to wall: an indicator of symmetry for functional positions such as plié and the ability to get the heels down during jumps.
- **Balance/proprioception:** star excursion balance test challenges both range in the lower limb and control; BIODEX single-leg athletic test; hop and hold for an assessment of control.
- **Muscle power:** jumping (height, distance, stam-

ina, symmetry, distance on single hop, distance on repeated hops, cross-overs, speed over distance, and so on; Optijump/force plate (if available).

- **Muscle strength:** knee, ankle extension/flexion isokinetics (if available).

'Functional' Testing

The ability to create adequate exit criteria through the various phases of an injury, as well as determining full return to dance, can be challenging. Understanding the functional requirements will form a fundamental part of any functional test. One example of this approach is the assessment of exit criteria of lumbo-pelvic to lower-limb injuries in ballet. Returning the heel to the ground when coming down from a rise en pointe or demi-pointe or a jump requires a systematic eccentric control sequence that starts at the foot. Initial contact is made with the forefoot and the foot is then lowered, with the heel, finally, being lowered eccentrically. Depending on the movement, as in a jump, the knee is then unlocked from an initial straight position, and at the same time the lowering is controlled through the glutes and posterior chain.

Designing an appropriate test to determine the dancer's ability to achieve this may be difficult if relying on objective measurements only. Being able to grade the quality of the control through the foot, and subsequently through the knees and hips, will give a better indication whether a dancer is fit to progress. One protocol being explored in ballet is the use of controlled rises and lowerings through the foot in a turn-out position to a predetermined metronome beat and 6 count. If this is successfully achieved, and symmetrical, the test is progressed to assess the dancer's ability to eccentrically control the heel drop by performing 'beats' on a heel rise in a turn-out position to a metronome. Again, symmetry is assessed. The dancer is instructed to work through the range with the lightest of touches of the heel to the floor, demonstrating their ability to eccentrically

control the movement as opposed to 'collapsing' to the floor.

If the first two stages are progressed satisfactorily, the final stage is the assessment of the jump/land mechanics. Careful evaluation of the landing mechanism looks for the heels to be lowered to the ground under control, without compensatory movements, and effective use of the glutes and knees. Again, this can be done at a pace determined by metronome. Symmetry between the affected and unaffected sides is a key indicator in making a decision about whether the dancer is fit to dance.

Further functional testing might include incremental participation in the stages of class (barre, centre and jumps), with additional work on lifting/partnering as relevant. This should be included with all dancers who are required to lift as part of their role, to ensure that they are safe to proceed.

Further Assessments

A challenging part of the return to play decision is related to strength and power endurance assessment. Dance may involve prolonged bouts of high-intensity intervals against longer work of a lower intensity. Using repeated strength (repeated lifts or rises) and power drills (jump box plyometric drills) with short recovery sessions can help inform the decisions. Additionally, evaluating chronic training load (as an exponent of exposure and training intensity) will help establish the suitability for return to a performance period, rather than just whether the dancer can perform the technical requirements for a single show.

An evaluation of the psychological readiness to return to full participation is also important. Anxiety and fear of further injury can be normal consequences of any injury. The use of exit criteria, incremental loading and physiological and functional or technical testing may inspire confidence and reduce anxiety for patients returning from injury, but some patients may benefit from additional input from a sports psychologist.

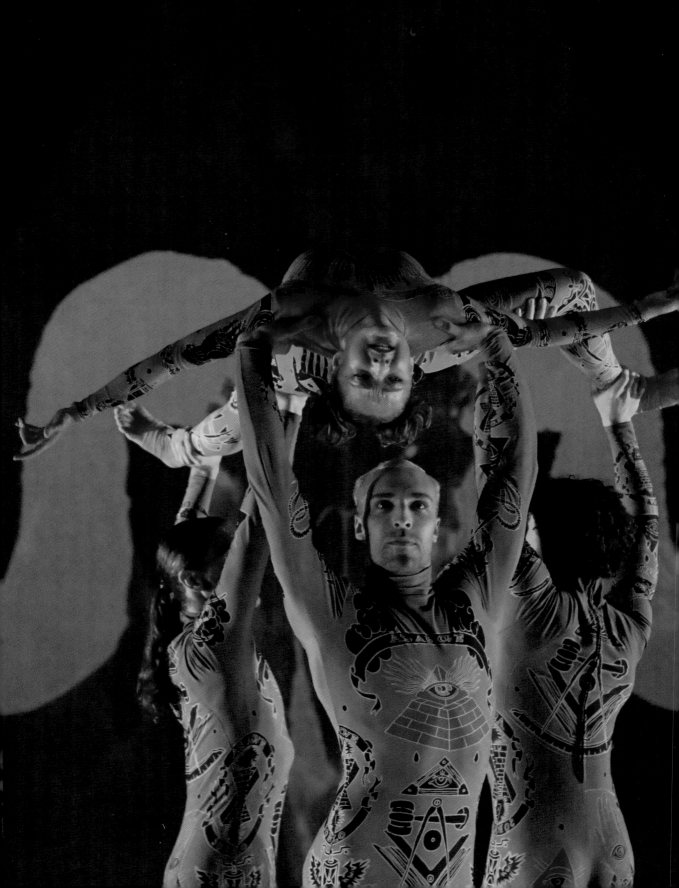

CHAPTER 6

HEAD AND NECK INJURIES

This chapter will explore the nature and incidence of injuries to the head and neck in dance. Although traumatic injuries are less frequent that overuse injuries, the trauma can have severe consequences and can be followed by concussion. Healthcare professionals need to pay particular attention to such injuries in all athletes, including dancers. Furthermore, the forces experienced on the neck by dancers, with lifting and turning, require a good understanding of the part of the attending clinician, in terms of the type of pathologies they may encounter.

HEAD

The reported incidence of head or face injuries in dance is low, but they do include concussion or head trauma. Traumatic brain injury is an area of critical importance in sports medicine and is covered by several international consensus statements. The latest, led by Paul McCory and an international expert panel in 2017, forms the basis for the discussion in this chapter. The work of the various international consensus authors has led to the evolution of the term 'sports-related concussion' to describe the immediate and transient symptoms of traumatic brain injury. The fifth International Conference on Concussion in Sport was clear in its indications:

Sport-related concussion (SRC) is a traumatic brain injury induced by biomechanical forces. Several common features that may be utilized in clinically defining the nature of a concussive head injury include:

- *SRC may be caused either by a direct blow to the head, face, neck or elsewhere on the body with an impulsive force transmitted to the head.*
- *SRC typically results in the rapid onset of short-lived impairment of neurological function that resolves spontaneously. However, in some cases, signs and symptoms evolve over a number of minutes to hours.*
- *SRC may result in neuropathological changes, but the acute clinical signs and symptoms largely reflect a functional disturbance rather than a structural injury and, as such, no abnormality is seen on standard structural neuroimaging studies.*
- *SRC results in a range of clinical signs and symptoms that may or may not involve loss of consciousness. Resolution of the clinical and cognitive features typically follows a sequential course. However, in some cases symptoms may be prolonged.*

Furthermore, the clinical signs and symptoms cannot be explained by drug, alcohol, or medication use, other injuries (such as cervical injuries, peripheral vestibular dysfunction, etc) or other comorbidities (e.g., psychological factors or coexisting medical conditions).

As can be seen from the features of sports-related concussion, it is important to recognize its possibility in dance and also to apply the same management process. The consensus statements for concussion make it clear that it is a potentially evolving injury, with any suspected concussion patient requiring immediate removal, to ensure the appropriate assessment of potentially rapidly changing clinical symptoms. The patient needs to undergo a thorough assessment in a distraction-free environment, by a healthcare professional familiar with concussion, using the standardized concussion assessment tool (SCAT 5, at time of publication). Concussion may be suspected if certain symptoms are present:

- somatic symptoms (for example, headache);
- cognitive symptoms (for example, the feeling of being 'in a fog') and/or emotional symptoms (for example, lability);
- physical signs, such as loss of consciousness, amnesia, neurological deficit;
- balance impairment (for example, gait unsteadiness);
- behavioural changes (for example, irritability);
- cognitive impairment (for example, slowed reaction times);
- sleep/wake disturbance (for example, somnolence, drowsiness)

It is important to note that, due to the changing nature of signs and symptoms in concussion, it may be necessary to undertake a number of evaluations over a period of time to confirm diagnosis. If in doubt, the symptoms should be treated as concussion until proven otherwise. Patients should not be left alone for at least a few hours post injury.

If SRC is suspected in a dancer, he or she should not be allowed to return to dance that day and the graduated full return to dance programme should be followed. Management of a patient with concussion involves a period of rest (24 to 48 hours), followed by gradual and progressive increasing activity/exercise in a safe environment. The level of intensity and duration may vary but it is important that the activity does not worsen the symptoms (physical and/or cognitive). The use of a static bike allows patients to measure output and increment exercise accordingly. When the dancer is clear of concussion symptoms (in the absence of pharmacological aids), the graduated return to dance increment protocol should be followed.

Patient response to each level needs careful assessment in relation to the return of symptoms or a change in technical ability compared with pre-concussion state.

The graduated return to dance protocol has a number of steps:

1. Physical and cognitive rest (24 to 48 hours).
2. Light aerobic activity (static cycle).
3. Technical coaching (barre, centre).
4. Class (barre, centre, jumps).
5. Rehearsal.
6. Return to performance.

The international consensus statement goes on to indicate the following:

Persistent symptoms following SRC should reflect failure of normal clinical recovery – that is, symptoms that persist beyond expected time frames (i.e. >10–14 days in adults and >4 weeks in children). Persistent symptoms do not reflect a single pathophysiological entity but describes a constellation of non-specific post-traumatic symptoms that may be linked to coexisting and/or confounding factors, which do not necessarily reflect on-going physiological injury to the brain).

If a dancer's symptoms worsen or persist, an onward referral to an appropriate specialist concussion or head injury unit is indicated.

NECK

Anatomy and Associated Pathology

The neck provides a multitude of critical functions in daily life, with a key role in supporting the weight of the head and protecting the spinal cord (and medulla oblongata). In dance, it has a vital role in the positioning of the head according to functional need and external stimuli, thereby impacting on balance.

There have been few reports of disc pathology in dance, and even fewer relating to the cervical region. It is the cervical component of the spine that is the most mobile, divided up into the occipital-atlantoaxial complex (C0-C1-C2), the middle cervical spine (C2-C5), and the lower cervical spine (C5-T1). Throughout the spine the vertebrae are connected and separated by intervertebral discs. Discs are comprised of a nucleus pulposus of Type II collagen fibres in an aqueous gel that is rich with proteoglycans, surrounded by concentric layers of collagen fibre bundles that form the annulus.

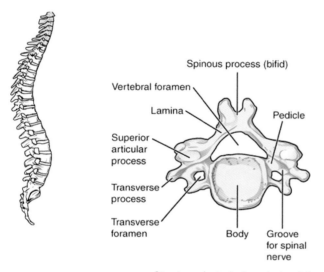

Structure of a typical cervical vertebra

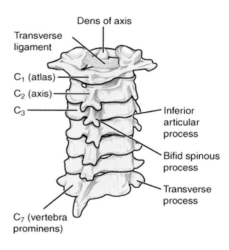

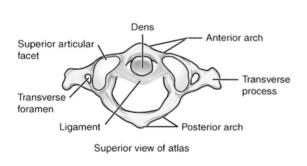

Superior view of atlas

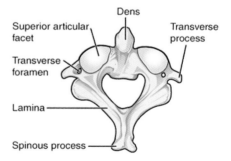

Superior view of axis

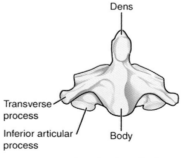

Anterior view of axis

Fig. 8 Anatomy of the cervical vertebrae.

Movement occurs through the various sections of the cervical spine, with C1 and 2 responsible for 50 per cent of rotation and 50 per cent of the flexion and extension occurring through the upper cervical spine.

Closely correlated with postural requirements in dance is the position of the upper and lower cervical spine in protraction and retraction. Dancers are known for their attention to a more upright posture moving. This utilizes a movement towards retraction, with an upper cervical flexed position and lower cervical extension, as opposed to a protracted posture, in which the upper cervical spine is extended and the lower cervical spine is flexed. The bony architecture plays a key role in the stability and movement of the spine. In the cervical region, the facets angle sits at around 45 degrees. Typically, the superior facet will glide over the inferior facet during movement. The facet joints are also surrounded by a strong capsule consisting of strong connective tissue.

There exists a potential for impingement and irritation of the facet region in dancers, given the rotational movements seen in fouettés and pirouettes, when they employ 'spotting' to prevent motion sickness. Aside from the rotational torque dancers may experience from turning drills, they may also be susceptible to acceleration/deceleration injuries with the rapid movements seen in some choreographies. The impact on muscle and ligamentous structures in this case needs to be considered seriously.

The neck is supported by deep and superficial layers of muscle. The role of the deep neck flexors, such as the longus capitus and longus colli, is important to dancers in postural holds and stabilization, and in the positioning of the head with turning. There are also layers of extensor muscles in the neck, including splenius capitus, splenius cervicus, spinalis, longissimus and semispinalius capitus. The deep muscle layers are associated with proprioception.

Another key aspect associated with dance is control of the breath, with an emphasis placed on diaphragmatic breathing. The diaphragm is innovated by the phrenic nerve, which originates at the C4 level. There is some evidence to demonstrate the impact of shallow breathing on various metabolic

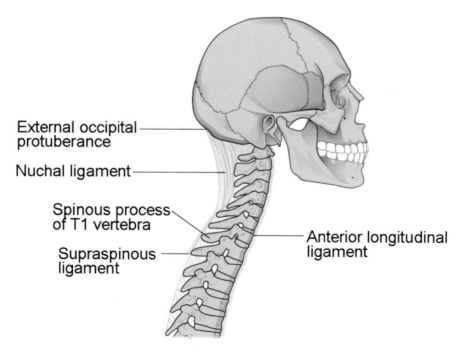

External occipital protuberance

Nuchal ligament

Spinous process of T1 vertebra

Supraspinous ligament

Anterior longitudinal ligament

Fig. 9 Anatomy of the cervical spine including ligaments.

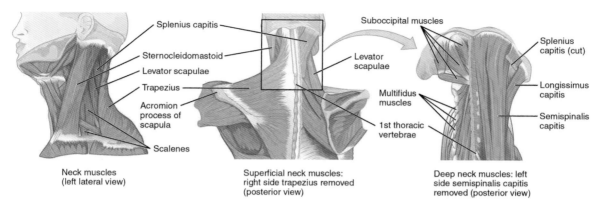

Splenius capitis

Sternocleidomastoid

Levator scapulae

Trapezius

Acromion process of scapula

Scalenes

Levator scapulae

Suboccipital muscles

Multifidus muscles

1st thoracic vertebrae

Splenius capitis (cut)

Longissimus capitis

Semispinalis capitis

Neck muscles (left lateral view)

Superficial neck muscles: right side trapezius removed (posterior view)

Deep neck muscles: left side semispinalis capitis removed (posterior view)

Fig. 10   Muscular anatomy of the neck.

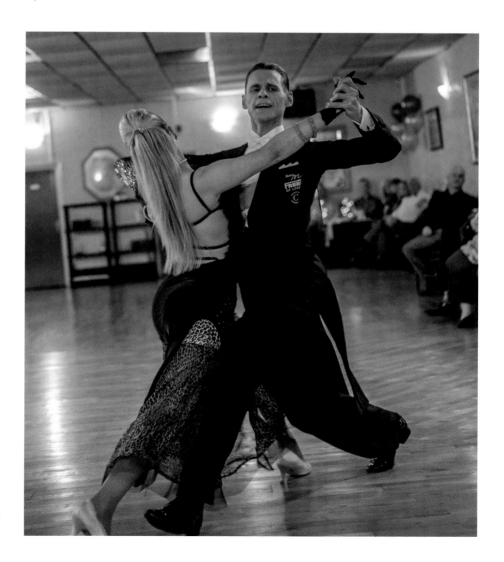

Photo 84   Ballroom posture. JACK BEALE

markers, ultimately resulting in changes in muscle tone and potentially creating a source of pain. The ability to maintain good stability and alignment of the neck is vital to support dancers who employ diaphragmatic breathing.

The blood supply for the posterior two-thirds of the brain is via the vertebral basilar artery, whose pathway is via the cervical vertebral foramina. Vertebral basilar artery insufficiency (VBAI) is typically identified with patients presenting with any of the '5 Ds': diplopia; dysathria; dysphagia; drop attacks; or dizziness. Additionally, symptoms may include nystagmus, nausea or tinnitus. Changes in muscle tone seen in dysfunctional biomechanics patterns can alter the position of the cervical segments. Changes to the alignment can also have an impact on blood supply and clinicians need to be aware of minor or transient symptoms associated with VBAI, and the role of hypertonic muscle changes in its presentation.

The incidence of cervical injuries in ballet has been reported as being between 0.47 and 0.53 injuries per 1000 hours. Most reported neck injuries originate from the cervical facet joints, with a reported incidence of 0.29–0.34 injuries per 1000 hours, with cervical muscle injuries also noted at 0.16–0.17 per 1000 hours of dancing. Onset varies from overloading in male dancers due to some choreographic lifts, via straining of cervical muscles through postural holds in ballroom dancers, through to stabilization of the head during floor work by contemporary dancers.

Differentiation between facet and muscle origin is important, as it will steer the early part of the management process. Cervical irritation often has a chemical origin and may respond to an anti-inflammatory approach in the early stage. Muscle-based injuries, although subject to some inflammatory responses, generally benefit from an approach based around muscle activation below the threshold of pain. In practice, both types of injury can present simultaneously and a pattern of dysfunctional biomechanical changes can result. It can begin with an initial irritation of the facet or surrounding structures, followed by a hypertonic muscle response, creating

a torticollis-type presentation. The increased tone creates a closing down of the facet, resulting in a smaller gap and therefore an approximation of the joints and surrounding soft tissue in simple movements such as cervical rotation or extension. Moreover, many spine-based pathologies are associated with the development of chronic pain patterns. Where appropriate, advice should be given regarding adequate analgesia to ensure normal movement patterns are established as soon as possible.

Discogenic pathologies are less prevalent in ballet populations but may be more of a problem for contemporary dancers undertaking floor work, where increased loads may be experienced through the head and neck. A questioning and examination of neurological symptoms are important in assessing the dancer's neck. Although unusual, the impact on the nerves from the neck, whether from a stinger or brachial plexus traction injury, or pressure causing a direct nerve referral, always needs to be considered. The use of a hand-held dynamometer to assess grip strength as a function of myotomes can provide an objective measure for both assessment and progress in patients with neurological deficits following neck injuries.

Rehabilitation of Neck Injuries in Dance

When designing a preventive or rehabilitation programme for dancers, there are a few key areas to consider. The role of the deep neck flexors is essential to good postural control. Good posture is of course synonymous with dance, but such control is an important foundation against sustaining neck injuries. A programme may begin with simple chin tucks in sitting, progressed to prone, to establish good postural control. This can then be extended to a prone head draw, where the chin tuck is maintained while moving from a dropped head position (in other words, a neck flex) to a position that resembles upright posture by extending the neck and not the head (Photos 85 and 86).

The work is then progressed to a four-way isometric strength training programme, which can be performed using a band. This is looped around the head in the desired direction and the dancer is then instructed to 'step away from the band', to increase the tension while maintaining a neutral position of the neck. This can be built up, from 10-second holds to 2-minute drills for sustained strength endurance. There are also various head harnesses available, usually used in sports such as motor racing and rugby. These generally have a rotational capacity and can be used to progress to spotting drills. 'Spotting' is the action that a dancer uses to prevent motion sickness when turning, by focusing on a single point through the turn and whipping the head round to spot it again (Photos 87 and 88).

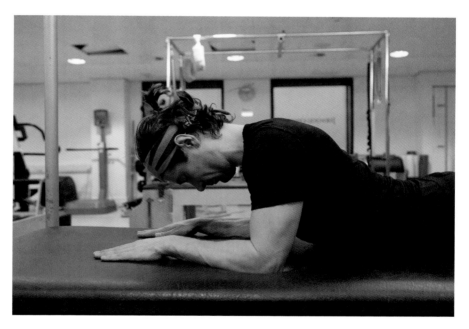

Photo 85 Start position for deep neck stabilizers.

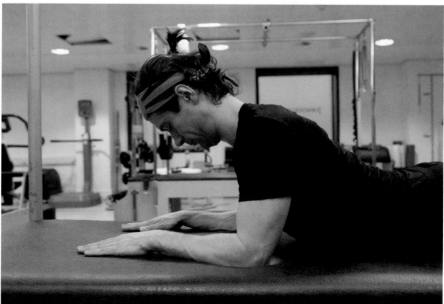

Photo 86 Finish position for deep neck stabilizers.

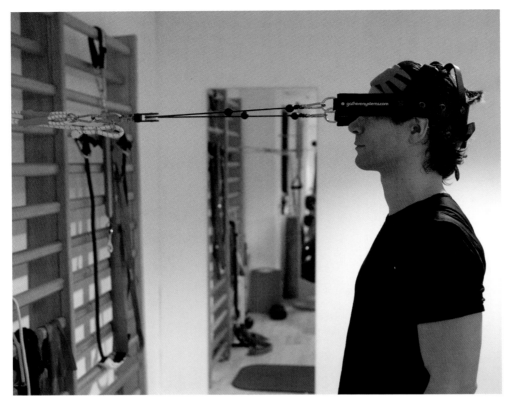

Photo 87
Standing
position for
deep neck
stabilizers.

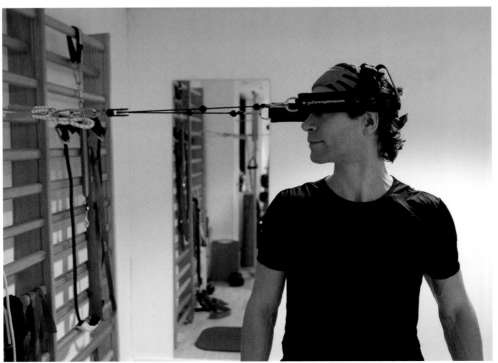

Photo 88
Spotting
position for
deep neck
stabilizers.

Table 1 Neck rehabilitation programme for dance.

Session 1 (2–4 weeks)	Time (sec)	Reps	Sets
Inhibition			
Foam roller releases	20–60		
Neuromuscular facilitation – isometric			
Scapula control/glenohumeral dissociation – prone wrist and elbow lift	8	8	2
Isometric 4-way neck holds	8	8	2
Isolate/strengthen			
Concentric seated chin tucks	10	2	
Eccentrics prone head drops with chin tuck	10	2	
Functional integration			
DG head harness isometric holds	8	8	2
DG head harness spotting	15	3	

As the dancer progresses through the rehabilitation process, the load and speed of the exercises should be progressed, ultimately concluding with turning and spotting drills at full functional (dance) speed. The inclusion of shoulder and thoracic stability and strength work is essential as part of a comprehensive programme. This work may include standard scapula stability drills, and rotator cuff exercises, as well as Palof press drills for thoracic stability.

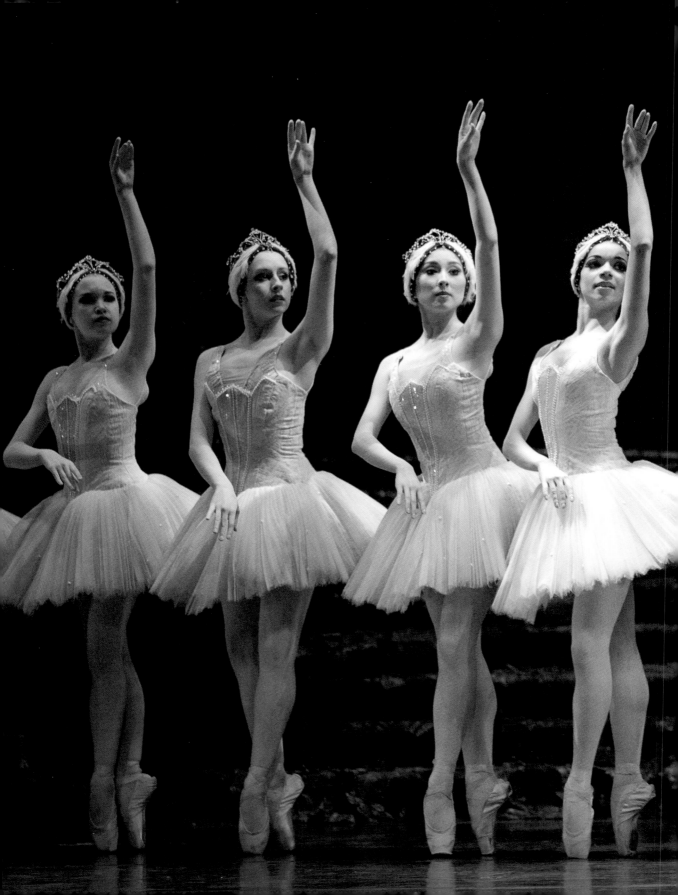

CHAPTER 7

INJURIES TO THE THORACIC REGION, SHOULDER, ARM AND HAND

This chapter will review the anatomy of the thoracic region, shoulder and arm, down to the hand and the wrist. Housing most of the body's vital organs, the thoracic region is a critical component of the protective cage of the chest, but it is also designed to facilitate the movement of the spine and ribs in everyday function. Dance challenges this function further, demanding extreme movement as well as a visible control of the appearance of breathing. The shoulder is a complex joint, with four 'articulations'. In view of the demands placed on the shoulder, with arm holds in second, fourth or fifth position,

lifting while partnering, and potential impact with floor work in contemporary choreography, it is not surprising that injuries are seen in this area. Although the prevalence of such injuries is less than that of those in the lower limb, their impact on performance ability is just as significant.

THORACIC REGION

Anatomy and Related Pathology

Unlike other sections of the spine, the thoracic component must incorporate its movement with

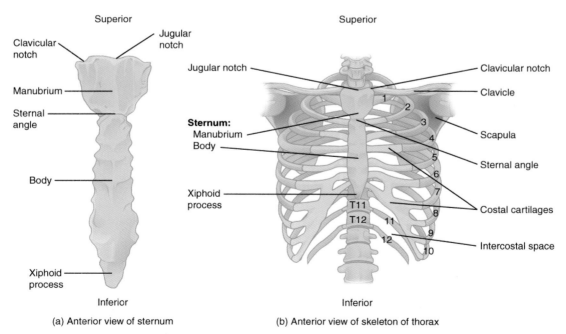

Fig. 11   Bony anatomy of the ribs and sternum.

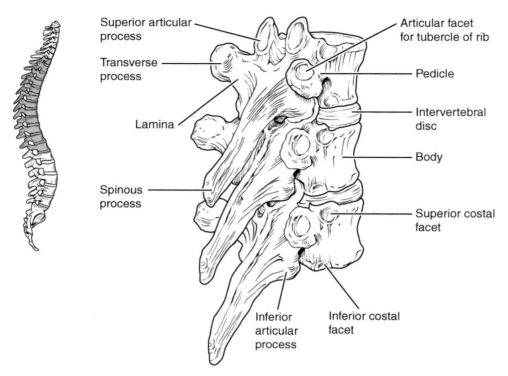

Fig. 12 Bony anatomy of the thoracic region.

the rib articulations. With the sternum positioned anteriorly there is less expected movement through this region. The thoracic spine is capable of flexion, extension, lateral flexion and axial rotation, often achieved via a coupling of movements. With the angle of the ribs, there is approximation of the ribs in lateral flexion.

When examining the thoracic region in dancers it is important to appreciate the importance of scapular position in lifting/partnering, postural holds and turning. There has been a higher reported incidence of thoracic region pain in male dancers. As part of the thoracic assessment it is important to look at the lifting technique of a male dancer. Some patterns show dancers failing to control load in the naturally kyphosis curvature of the thoracic spine positions and 'giving' in at the thoracic region, which may cause facet joint stiffness or irritation.

Identifying the potential presence of a thoracic scoliosis is important, as it has implications for rotation and scapula positioning (typically with a 'winging' scapula noted on the scoliotic side). Although

it is particularly relevant when examining spinal pain in adolescent dancers, the impact of conditions such as Scheuermann's disease and a lack of thoracic mobility in skeletally mature patients also needs to be appreciated. Pain may originate from end plate and Schmorls nodes regions. Furthermore, any restriction in rotation through the thoracic region, and a subsequent increased or hyperlordotic compensation in the lumbar region, with added rotational torque in twisting or extension movements, needs to be carefully examined in adult dancers with thoracic or lumbar pain and a past medical history, including Scheuermann's disease.

Challenges to the Thoracic Region in Partnering

It is important to recognize the fact that the role of a female dancer during partnering or pas de deux is not passive, but requires a strong spinal and trunk posture. Core trunk strength is very important in a female dancer. Additionally, a lack of technical ability in the male partner, particularly in terms of hand placement and grip strength on the female dancer, can contribute to pain in the thoracic region, most notably around rib articulations.

In the case of sprained or irritated rib articulations, early-stage management may include strapping to minimize the 'bucket handle' movement of the ribs and reduce irritation at the thoracic articulation. Middle-stage rehabilitation should focus on improving core and trunk strength, while end-stage rehabilitation might include technical support and even a partner, to ensure hand placement and grip strength in lifts are appropriate.

Table 2 Initial rehabilitation programme for thoracic injuries in dance.

Session 1 (2–4 weeks)	Time (sec)	Reps	Sets
Inhibition			
Foam roller releases	20– 60	NA	1–2
Neuromuscular facilitation/isometric			
Scapula control/glenohumeral dissociation – prone wrist and elbow lift	8	8	2
Isometric Pallof press	8	8	2
Isolate/strengthen/muscle endurance			
Concentric			
Swiss ball reverse glut ham raise	slow	10–12	2–4
Eccentrics			
Swiss ball supine trunk rotations	slow	10–12	2–4
Functional integration			
Plank: 3-point hold (alternate single limb lift)	5	8	2
Resisted trunk rotations in third (arm) position	30	1	1

Table 3 Mid-stage rehabilitation programme for thoracic injuries in dance.

Session 2 (2 weeks)	Time (sec)	Reps	Sets
Inhibition			
Foam roller releases	20–60	NA	1–2
Neuromuscular facilitation – isometric			
Standing scapula control/glenohumeral dissociation	8	8	2
Isometric trunk holds (front, back, sides)	8	8	2
Isolate/strengthen/muscle endurance			
Concentric			
Swiss ball trunk extensions	slow	10–12	2–4
Rotator cuff – arm at side	slow	10–12	2–4
Eccentrics			
Pallof press with controlled rotation		10–12	2–4
Functional integration			
Floor swimmers	NA	6	2–4
Incline chest pulls	NA	6	2–4
Reach and pull	NA	6	2–4

Table 4   End-stage rehabilitation programme for thoracic injuries in dance.

Session 3 (2 weeks)	Time (sec)	Reps	Sets
Inhibition			
Foam roller releases	20–60		
Neuromuscular facilitation/isometric			
Wall Blackmanns – T,Y,W isometric holds	20	2	1
Wall arm slides	slow	8	2
Isolate/strengthen			
Concentric			
Back flys (suspension cable)		6	4–6
Rotator cuff – shoulder 90deg		6	4–6
Eccentrics			
Swiss ball supine metronome		12	2
Functional integration			
Press-up plus – lift, rotate, extend		6	2–4
Face pulls with external rotation at shoulder	15–18	2–3	
Single-leg Romanian dead lift		15–18	2–3

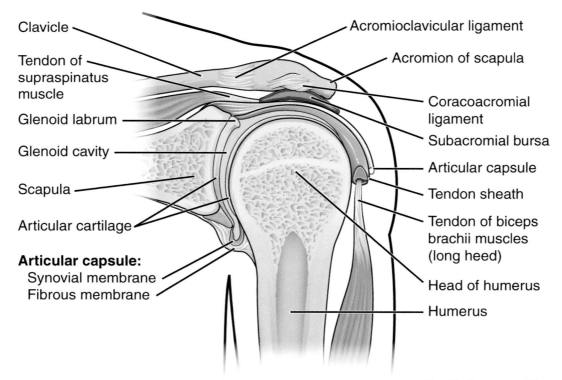

Fig. 13   Anatomy of the glenohumeral joint.

SHOULDER

Anatomy and Related Pathology

The shoulder joint is comprised of four joints: the glenohumeral, acromioclavicular and sternoclavicular, with the scapulothoracic a functional rather than true joint. This unique arrangement provides a remarkable range of movement, but the downside of this extended range of movements can be a compromise in stability.

The sternoclavicular joint provides the articulation with the rest of the skeleton, so there is an increased demand on the surrounding muscles to create stability for the shoulder girdle. Although subluxations of the sternoclavicular joint can occur in contact sports such as rugby, they are rare in dance. The disc and costoclavicular ligament play a key role in reducing forces through the joint. Pain around the sternoclavicular region has been reported in dancers following glenohumeral ligament reconstruction, where the alteration in biomechanics can affect the normal rotary and translator movement that occurs here. This may also be seen in dancers presenting with a protracted shoulder, increasing the compressive forces through the joint and disc. Occasionally, these dysfunctional biomechanical changes may manifest in irritation of the sternoclavicular disc. A T1 weighted MRI will help examine the chondral surface, while a T2 MRI sequence is useful to confirm whether the loading has extended to the surrounding bone tissue with the presence of a high signal return there.

Clavicular fractures have been reported rarely in dance. At the other end of the clavicle is the acromioclavicular joint. Like the sternoclavicular joint, this is protected by a fibrocartilage disc and supported by ligaments and a weak capsule. There is a high reported prevalence of trauma to the acromioclavicular joint in contact sports, but the prevalence of such injuries is low in dance. The acromioclavicular joint plays a key role in tipping as well as internal and external rotation. Failure of the acromion to posteriorly tip during elevation and flexion of the arm to more than 60 degrees can lead to subacromial impingement. Although subacromial impingement may be more descriptive of symptomology rather than pathology based, there is a potential sequalae that may result in greater pathological structural consequence. Repeated dysfunctional or poorly tolerated loading of the rotator cuff muscles, like supraspinatus, may result in a tendinosis presentation. The consequence of this is to reduce the efficiency of the muscle in performing its stabilizing function of the shoulder mechanics, including humeral head migration. This may result in multi-directional instability as well as impingement risk in the subacromial space. An even greater risk may be the risk of damage to the labrum, or subluxation or dislocation

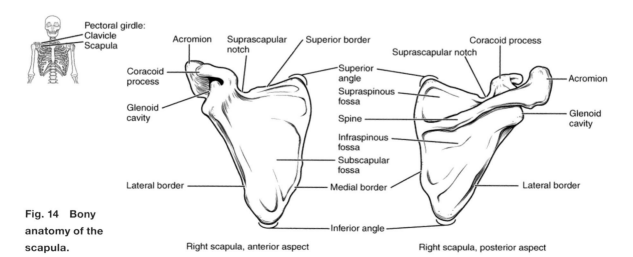

Fig. 14 Bony anatomy of the scapula.

Pectoral girdle:
Clavicle
Scapula

Acromion
Suprascapular notch
Superior border
Coracoid process
Suprascapular notch

Coracoid process
Glenoid cavity
Lateral border

Superior angle
Supraspinous fossa
Spine
Infraspinous fossa
Subscapular fossa
Medial border
Inferior angle

Acromion
Glenoid cavity
Lateral border

Right scapula, anterior aspect

Right scapula, posterior aspect

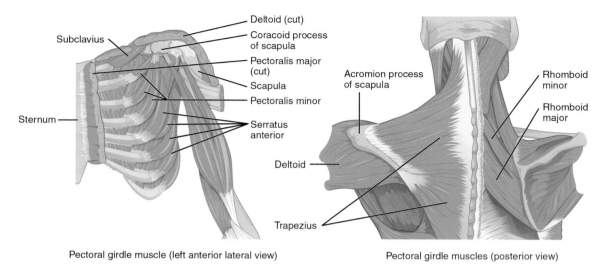

Pectoral girdle muscle (left anterior lateral view)

Pectoral girdle muscles (posterior view)

Fig. 15 Muscular anatomy of the shoulder girdle.

of the humeral head. In view of the impact of the arm positions in many balletic and other dance poses, it is vital for the clinical practitioner in dance to have an understanding of the underlying mechanics and potential patho-biomechanical changes.

Movement of the scapula against the posterior thoracic wall is key to achieving may dance-related functions and poses a related injury risk. Protraction and retraction of the clavicle at the sternoclavicular joint and rotation of the acromioclavicular joint facilitate the tipping seen through the scapulothoracic joint. Assessment of the position of the scapula at rest and through movement is important as an assessment of the neuromuscular control of the shoulder complex. Shoulder biomechanics can be assessed using the SICK mnemonic: S, Scapula malposition; I, Inferior medial scapular winging; C, Coracoid pain; and K, scapular dysKinesis.

Because of the way the shoulder articulations connect with the rest of the axial skeleton, there is a great dependency on the rotator cuff group of muscles (supraspinatus, infraspinatus, teres minor and subscapularis), and the surrounding muscles, to provide dynamic stability of the shoulder complex. This is achieved as a force coupling effect with various muscles in the region. The middle and lower portion of the trapezius muscle, along with the serratus anterior, are important in maintaining the scapular position flush to the posterior chest wall. The presence of inferior scapular winging indicates a potential deficiency in these groups. The 'balance' between tight anterior muscles like the pectoralis major, which attach to the coracoid process with the posterior shoulder, form an important part of the assessment and management planning. A painful coracoid could be linked with a tight pectoralis major.

There is a lower reported incidence of shoulder injuries in female dancers compared with male dancers. Both genders are required to position their arms in an abducted and elevated position in sustained holds, requiring the shoulder complex to maintain scapular positioning. However, lifting requires particularly good strength and stability in male dancers, alongside technique. The noted higher prevalence of hypermobility in dancers (both acquired and benign) can point to reduced stability, resulting in shoulder injuries.

The highest prevalence of shoulder injuries reported in ballet is related to subacromial impingement. In many overhead sports, such injuries have been associated with a restriction of internal rota-

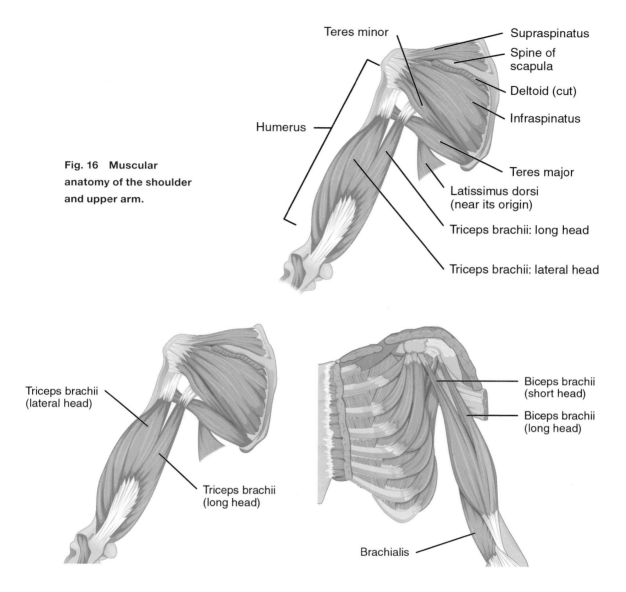

Teres minor

Supraspinatus

Spine of scapula

Deltoid (cut)

Infraspinatus

Humerus

Teres major

Latissimus dorsi (near its origin)

Triceps brachii: long head

Triceps brachii: lateral head

Fig. 16 Muscular anatomy of the shoulder and upper arm.

Triceps brachii (lateral head)

Triceps brachii (long head)

Biceps brachii (short head)

Biceps brachii (long head)

Brachialis

tion or glenohumeral internal rotation deficit (GIRD). While this does occur in dancers, it tends to be related to the impingement of supraspinatus, due to a failure of the scapula to posteriorly tip and sit flush to the posterior chest wall while the arm is abducted and elevated.

It is important to differentiate between an impingement of supraspinatus and a tendinosis adaptation. In this case, even traumatic episodes with a defined inciting event warrant careful appreciation of scapula control through movement and conditioning.

to support optimal scapula mechanics. Given the nature of dance, superior as well as posterior labral tears have been reported. These can be both traumatic or through overuse and may present as an acute episode, with an inciting event, or as a chronically unstable shoulder.

Labral damage does not always necessitate surgical intervention. Compliance with a comprehensive rehabilitation and conditioning programme can support the shoulder and allow dancers to return to full function without limitation. As with all injuries, this still requires careful monitoring, to ensure reoccurrence or subsequent injuries do not result from a lack of structural integrity of the shoulder labrum. Ultimately, increased mobility or lack of stability and strength may lead to subluxation or dislocation of the shoulder. In these instances, the surgical option is usually required, but it is important to balance the risk of future episodes against any lack of range that may be seen post-operatively.

Rehabilitation of Shoulder Pathology in Dance

Rehabilitation of a dancer's shoulders needs to consider the functional range requirements of dance and balance them against the stability and strength needed. In the early stages of rehabilita-

tion, whether post-injury or post-surgery, range may seem an obvious primary objective. Indeed, it is true that structural restrictions in the shoulder's range of movement, for example potential capsular restriction, needs to be evaluated against the presence of a protective hypertonic rotator cuff response. As this remains a challenging differentiation, it would be pertinent to focus primarily on the restoration of optimal scapula thoracic patterning through a programme of neuromuscular control of the scapula muscles. This may entail isometric contraction of the internal and external rotators of the shoulder in elevated and abduction positions.

One fundamental requirement in the successful implementation of a neuromuscular or core control

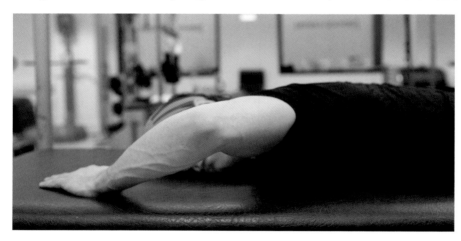

Photo 89   Scapula stabilization with prone elbow lift.

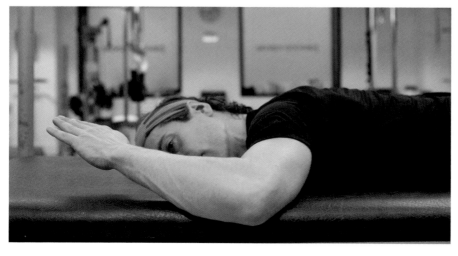

Photo 90   Scapula stabilization with prone wrist lift.

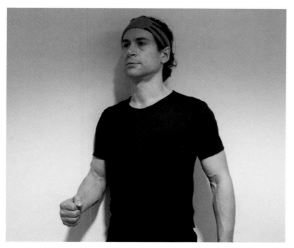

Photo 91   Scapula stabilization in standing starting position.

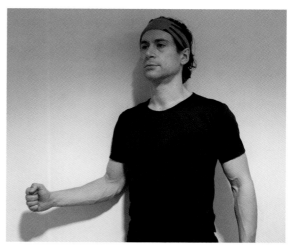

Photo 92   Scapula stabilization in standing finishing position.

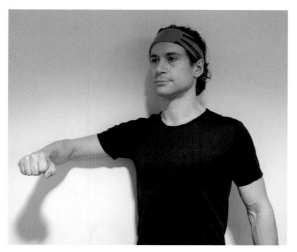

Photo 93   Scapula stabilization in standing and abduction starting position.

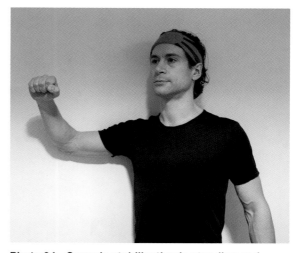

Photo 94   Scapula stabilization in standing and abduction finishing position.

programme is the achievement of movement without compensation. In the case of shoulder rehabilitation, this entails the ability to maintain an isometric contraction of the internal or external rotators without a noted increase in upper trapezius activation or elevation of the shoulder girdle. As the dancer moves through the rehabilitation process, this may be progressed from prone isometric drills to standing, and finally to maintaining scapula positioning through turns and lifts (Photos 89–94).

Utilizing the Hybrid Intervention Model (HIM) programme design, any identified strength deficit may be addressed in the early stage through isometric or inner range rotator cuff strength work. A SICK assessment of a scapula will also steer the programme design, identifying whether middle and lower trapezius and serratus anterior activation work is also required. In the presence of a winging scapula, this may indicate strength work. With scapular dyskinesis, the focus may be more on motor pattern work. In clinical practice, there are usually components of both.

Once achieved, this can be progressed into resolving any remaining range deficit, while developing baseline slow-twitch strength and additional glenohumeral stability. Through the rehabilitation process, this is progressed to strength through the full available range, then to more dynamic drills, engaging faster-twitch responses including closed- and open-chain drills such as plyometric press-ups and ball-trampette rebound exercises. This is further progressed to include the development of strength endurance and power endurance.

End-stage specificity needs to be added when

CASE STUDY 1: REHABILITATION POST-SURGICAL INTERVENTION FOR LABRAL DAMAGE

A professional male contemporary dancer had a superior labral tear that failed to resolve with conservative treatment and subsequently underwent surgical repair. Timelines for return to dance were determined using both biological timelines and conditioning timelines. Given a suspected sequalae of rotator cuff dysfunction leading to an initial presentation of subacromial impingement,

Table 5   Rehabilitation programme for a superior labral tear.

WEEK	1	2	3–4	5–8	9–12	13–16	17+
Unload and core/legs							
Support sling	•	•	•				
Isometric shoulder (abd, add, int, ext) 3x10sec holds each hour		•	•				
Gentle shoulder movement (pendular, elevate to max. shoulder height – not extreme int/ext)			•	•			
Static bike cycle session (focus on fitness and muscle endurance in the absence of class)			•	•	•		
Core session 1 as tolerated			•	•	•		
Leg session 1 training as tolerated			•				
ROM/strength							
Active (short levers) and active assisted ROM (all directions)				•	•		
Passive physiological mobilization of the shoulder				•	•		
Leg session 2 training as tolerated				•	•		
Shoulder session 1				•	•		
Proprioception/functional strength							
Shoulder session 2						•	•
Core session 2						•	•
Technical coaching						•	•
Shoulder session 3							•
Functional integration							
Class						•	
Rehearsal							•
Performance							•

enough range, strength and stability has been achieved to provide protection for the shoulder. End-stage rehab may include postural holds during turning/pirouettes and the use of water-filled Swiss balls in lifting drills, to mimic a partner's movements during lifts. Contemporary dancers aiming to do floor work need to ensure that they have undertaken plyometric work, and have developed sufficient closed-chain strength to support their artistic requirements. Within the functional integration components of the rehabilitation process, there must be a progression to postural holds and maintaining optimal scapula positioning during barre, centre and jumping and lifting drills.

there was increased emphasis to address this within the rehabilitation programme. This involved isolated rotator cuff strength work and scapula stability drills.

The programme was designed to facilitate the rehabilitation process as well as consider the functional requirements of the dancer and a return to lifting and floor work. The specific exercises referenced are given in Tables 6–8.

(continued overleaf)

Table 6   Core exercises.

	Reps	Sets	Rest
Core session 1			
Abductor isometric squeeze (0/45/90deg)	3×6–10sec hold/range	3	6–10sec
Sahrmann heel taps	8–12	3	30sec
Resisted clams	8–12	3	30sec
Side-lying clock	8–12	3	30sec
Prone hip extension	8–12	3	30sec
Core session 2			
Swiss ball prone/supine lateral roll outs	8–12/position	2	30sec
Swiss ball bridge	8–12	3	30sec
Swiss ball jack knife	8–12	3	30sec
Swiss ball sprinter's drill	8–12	3	30sec

Table 7   Leg exercises.

	Reps	Sets	Rest
Leg session 1			
Resistance band ankle push and pull through	15–25	4	30sec
Reformer squats	15–26	4	30sec
Reformer squats	15–26	4	30sec
Leg session 2			
Body weight squats	8–12	3	30sec
Body weight lateral squats	8 -12	3	30sec

CASE STUDY 1: REHABILITATION POST-SURGICAL INTERVENTION FOR LABRAL DAMAGE *(continued)*

Table 8   Shoulder exercises.

	Reps	Sets	Rest
Shoulder session 1 (1–2 daily)			
Wall Blackmanns (5/7, 9/3, 11/1)	3×5sec hold per level	3	30sec
Wall scapula setting (arm at close to 90deg int rot)	5–8	2	10sec
Wall scapula setting (arm at 30deg ext)	5–8	2	10sec
Wall windscreen wiper (10–2)	30sec	2	10sec
Pinch and push in side-lying	5–8	3	30sec
Side-lying ext rotation	8–12	3	30sec
Side-lying abduction to parallel	8–12	3	30sec
Wall-press shoulder retraction/protraction	8–12	3	30sec
Rotator cuff in standing (int, ext rotation)	8–12 per movement	3	30sec
Floor angels	10–15	3	10sec
Shoulder session 2 (am) daily			
Swimmers (prone on a bench)	5–8	4	10sec
Renegade press-up with row, rotate and lift	4–6	6	30sec
BOSU ball press (4-point kneeling or plank)	12–15	2	30sec
Swiss ball plank shoulder circles	6/direction	3	30sec
Scapula lunges	10–12	3	30sec
Shoulder session 2 (pm) 3–4x week			
Bent-over row	4–6	6	30sec
Shoulder shrugs and roll	4–6	6	30sec
Shoulder abduction (cable or resistance band)	4–6	6	30sec
Arnold press (body weight or light load)	4–6	6	30sec
Bench press	4–6	6	30sec
Bicep curls	4–6	6	30sec
Triceps extensions	4–6	6	30sec
Dips	4–6	6	30sec
Lat pull-downs/assisted chin-ups	4–6	6	30sec
Shoulder session 3 (alt with session 2 pm)			
Swiss water ball lift	15–18	3–4	30sec
Single-arm press and step	15–18	3–4	30sec
In-line wood chop cable	15–18	3–4	30sec
Dynamic wood chop	15–18	3–4	30sec
Supine catch and throw (progress to trampette)	15–18	3–4	30sec
Swiss ball crawlers prone (2 balls)	6/arm	2	30sec

ELBOW, WRIST AND HAND

Anatomy and Associated Pathology

A modified hinge joint, the elbow is made up of the articulations between the humerus proximally and the radius and ulna, allowing movement through 0 degrees extension (although dancers with hypermobility may present with hyperextension greater than 10 degrees) to around 135 degrees flexion, with a small amount of axial rotation through the ulna. The elbow is supported by the medial and lateral collateral ligaments and encased on a weak capsule.

Movement into flexion is created by the brachialis, biceps and brachioradialis that cross the joint anteriorly, while extension is as a result of the triceps and anconeus muscles that cross the joint posteriorly. The radioulnar joints link proximally and inferiorly to allow rotation in pronation at around 70 degrees, and supination at around 80 degrees through the actions of the pronator teres, pronator quadratus, biceps brachii and supinator. From a dance perspective, a functional range of around 100 degrees between pronation and supination is needed.

The wrist is a complex region, comprising the two long bones of the forearm (radius and ulna) that make up the distil radial ulna joint (DRUJ) and the eight carpal bones. These then lead into the metacarpals of the hand. The radiocarpal joint allows flexion, extension, radial and ulna deviation as well as circumduction movements. These are facilitated through accessory movement and in particular gliding through the midcarpal joints. The wrist is supported by a fibrous capsule, which is thickened by intrinsic ligaments that connect the carpal bones. On the dorsal side, these are the scapholunate ligament (dorsal segment); lunotriquetral ligament (dorsal segment); scaphotriquetral ligament; scaphotrapeziotrapezoid ligament. On the palmar side, they are the scapholu-nate ligament (palmar segment), lunotriquetral ligament (palmar segment), scaphotriquetral ligament, radial collateral ligament, ulnar collateral ligament, scaphotrapeziotrapezoid ligament, and interosseous ligaments. Extrinsic ligaments attach the carpal bones to the radius and ulna and include on the dorsal side the dorsal radiotriquetral ligament (DRT) and dorsal ulnotriquetral ligament. On the palmar side, they are the radioscaphocapitate ligament (RSC), radiolunotriquetral ligament, radioscapholunate ligament (RSL), short radiolunate ligament (SRL), ulnolunate ligament (UL) and palmar ulnotriquetral ligament (UT).

Movement is achieved with the flexor group of muscles (flexor carpi ulnaris, flexor carpi radialis and palmaris longus) and extensor group (extensor carpi radialis longus, extensor carpi radialis brevis and extensor carpi ulnaris).

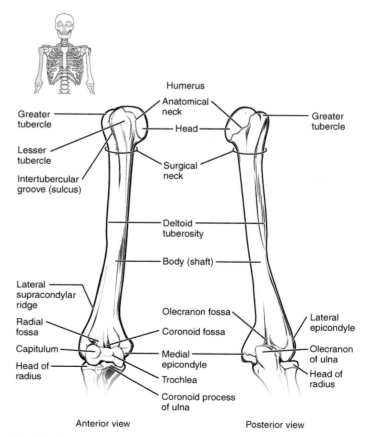

Humerus

Anatomical neck

Greater tubercle

Head

Greater tubercle

Lesser tubercle

Surgical neck

Intertubercular groove (sulcus)

Deltoid tuberosity

Body (shaft)

Lateral supracondylar ridge

Radial fossa

Capitulum

Head of radius

Olecranon fossa

Coronoid fossa

Medial epicondyle

Trochlea

Coronoid process of ulna

Lateral epicondyle

Olecranon of ulna

Head of radius

Anterior view

Posterior view

Fig. 17   Bony anatomy of the upper arm and elbow.

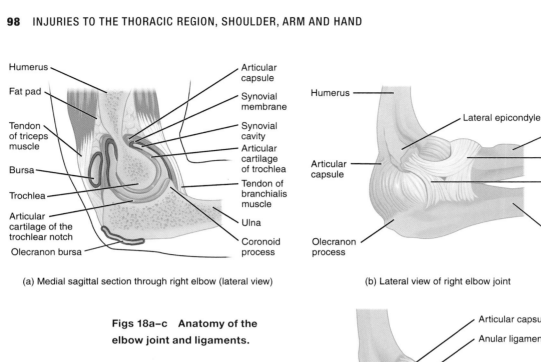

(a) Medial sagittal section through right elbow (lateral view)

(b) Lateral view of right elbow joint

Figs 18a–c Anatomy of the elbow joint and ligaments.

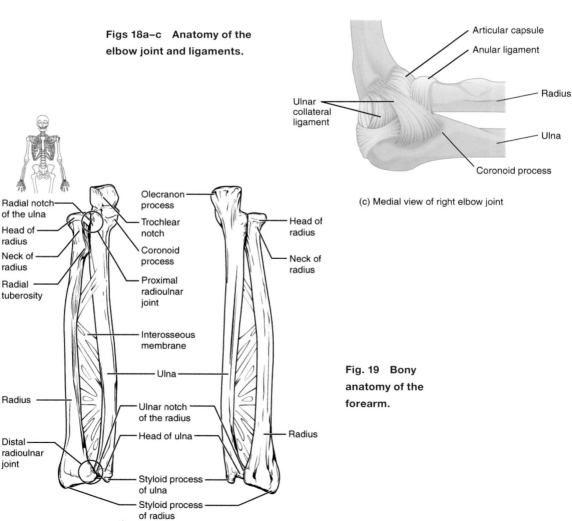

(c) Medial view of right elbow joint

Fig. 19 Bony anatomy of the forearm.

Fig. 20   Bony anatomy of the wrist and hand.

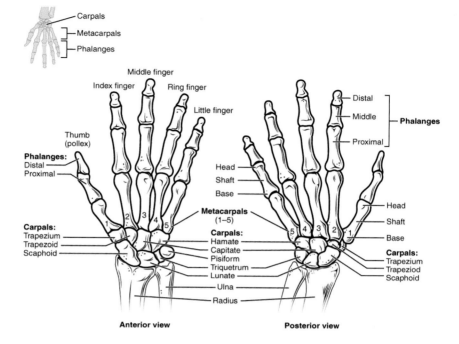

Anterior view

Posterior view

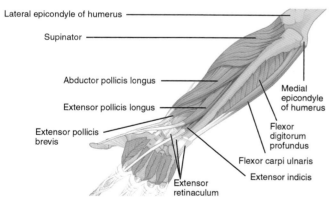

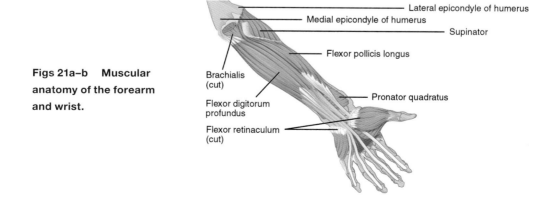

Figs 21a–b   Muscular anatomy of the forearm and wrist.

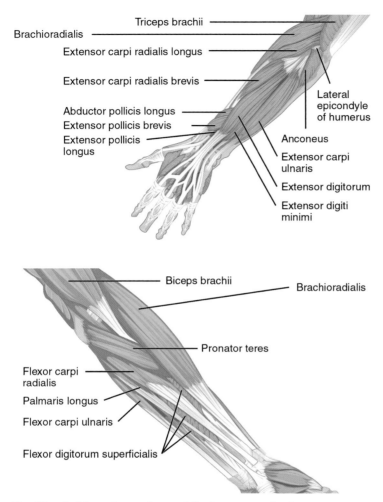

Figs 21c–d   Muscular anatomy of the forearm and wrist.

ing, however the realignment of a dislocated elbow entails the longitudinal distraction of the forearm at 45 degrees of elbow flexion. Assessment of vascular compromise pre- and post-alignment is critical.

A fall on to an outstretched hand may result in a fractured radial head or neck or distal humerus. Compressive trauma may also result in damage to the proximal humeroradial or humeroulnar joints. A fall on to an extended elbow can result in a dislocation or fracture of the coronoid process. The path of the ulna nerve through the posterior elbow may also be susceptible to compressive trauma. Male dancers involved in partnering may present with common flexor or extensor origin tendon problems. The prevalence of tendinopathy has been associated with complementary training and strength work in the gym rather than being specific to dance. A fall from height may result in bone injury, such as a supracondylar, olecranon or radial head fracture. Given the high complication rates of these regions, early investigation and orthopaedic opinion are recommended.

Prevalence, Diagnosis and Management

There is a low prevalence of elbow injuries in ballet, and contemporary dancers have reported a similarly low incidence of such injuries. Elbow injuries in dance are typically associated with floor work and are more traumatic in nature. Falls from height can result in posterior dislocations of the elbow. Given the high risk of compromise in this case, it is important to realign anatomically as soon as possible, with appropriate checks via x-rays to establish alignment and bony injury status. Detailed pre-hospital care is beyond the scope of this book and needs to be part of any clinician's on-going postgraduate train-

There is also a lower prevalence of wrist and hand injuries in dance, with carpal row sprains typically reported, including piso-triquetal and lunate triquetal sprains. In view of the nature of floor work, with some dancers it is important to exclude damage to the scaphoid, scaphoid-lunate ligament and triangular fibrocartilage complex (TFCC) regions. Watson's test, for scaphoid-lunate disruption or dorsiflexion/ulna deviation with rotation and overpressure for the TFCC, is useful to steer management to the appropriate structures. In contemporary dancers who are subject to repeated trauma as a result of floor work, and who report chronic wrist pain, it is important to assess the lunate, to exclude Kienbocks disease or avascular necrosis of the lunate.

A fall from height is also a potential mechanism to cause a fracture to the distal radius or ulna. The relationship between the base of the ulna and the TFCC requires careful assessment, to establish the stability of the distal radio-ulna joint (DRUJ).

Partnering is highly technical, requiring good shoulder strength and control, as well as grip strength, to ensure the partner is supported. The use of hand-held dynamometry can be a useful adjunct in determining any asymmetrical deficits between the affected and unaffected sides in regard to non-specific grip strength. If utilized as part of a screening process, it may enable better advice as to what strength may be required to reduce the risk of injury to the arm, elbow and wrist in dancers. Gender, technical ability and dance genre also need to be respected in such screening.

Rehabilitation of wrist sprains needs to take into account a dancer's need to extend the wrist fully for certain aspect of partnering and floor work. Residual stiffness sometimes seen in chronic wrist sprains may benefit from physiotherapy intervention, with a focus on restoring range of movement while developing the functional strength.

Hand- and finger-based injuries are uncommon in dance compared with other sports, but genre and choreography can have an impact on their incidence. One relatively rare condition is De Quervain's tenosynovitis, which should be considered when a patient presents with a positive Finkelstein's test. Potential causes of this in dance might include sword work on stage in pieces such as *Romeo and Juliet*. Less prevalent is intersection syndrome, in which the abductor pollicis longus and extensor pollicis brevis cross the extensor carpi radialis. Dancers who partner are at risk of ulna collateral ligament sprains of the first metacarpal phalangeal joint, either from the thumb being forced through contact with the partner or pulled when caught in part of a costume. In most sports, a supportive brace may be applied in the early stages, followed by strapping through early stage competition, but this is often restricted in dance. With costumes playing an integral part of the story-telling, the use of simple thumb strapping may be prohibited on stage.

Floor-based choreography, seen more commonly in contemporary work, and partnering, can both introduce a greater risk of finger injury. These may include fractures to the metacarpal or phalanx bones.

A basic understanding of the complex anatomy of the finger is important in assisting the attending healthcare practitioner to diagnose and manage pathology. Movement occurs through the metacarpal phalangeal joints, distal and proximal interphalangeal joints. It is important to appreciate the presence and role of the volar plates, comprised of the collateral ligaments attaching to dense fibrous connective tissue. Due to the movement required at the joints, this tissue has an ability to 'concertina' with finger flexion. This property of the volar plate is important when considering options available in the presence of damage or tears to it. Although it is not common in dance, disruption of the volar plate through hyperextension of the finger or dislocation requires early intervention. In the initial stages, splinting may help avoid a flexion deformity. Splinting may need to be serial, with reducing degrees of flexion. Damage to the central slip (part of the dorsal extensor tendon that extends the proximal interphalangeal joint) is often seen with volar plate injuries.

Direct impact to the distal phalanx can result in a forced flexion injury to the extensor tendon, resulting in a 'mallet' finger. This may be due to tendon rupture or a small avulsion fracture. Again, splinting as an immediate intervention could be considered. Less common in dance is damage to the flexor tendon (jersey finger), where the finger is then held in an extended position. An orthopaedic opinion should be sought if damage to tendons is suspected. Damage to the collateral ligaments is also possible with partnering. 'Buddy' splinting the adjacent finger is usually effective during the initial healing phase but this may need to be reviewed at a later stage.

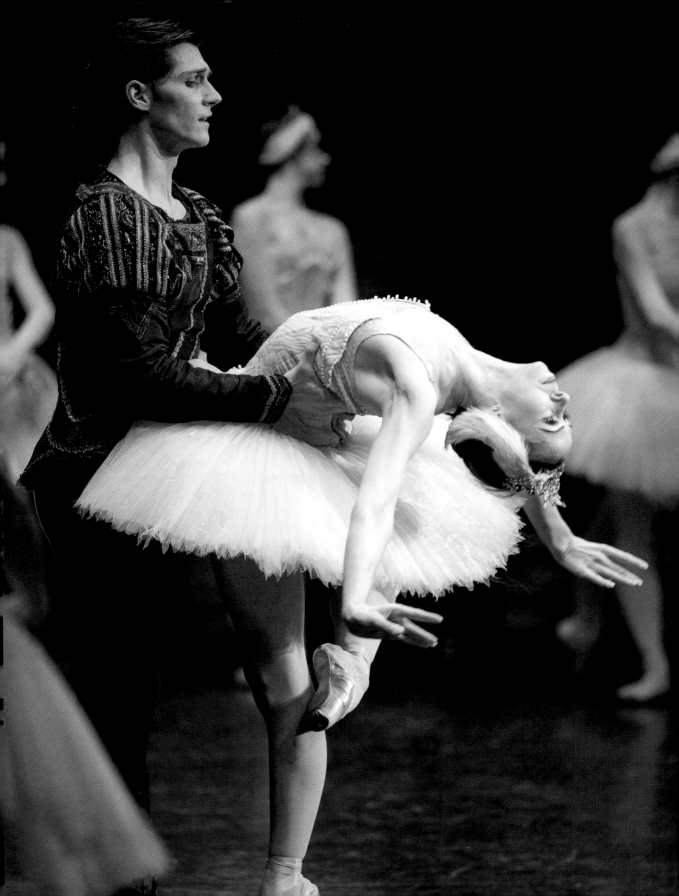

CHAPTER 8

LUMBAR, PELVIC, HIP AND GROIN INJURIES

In normal daily function, the lumbo-pelvic region serves as a major torque convertor, with ground reaction forces working cephalically and axial forces caudally with any lifting activity. The bony morphology and supporting ligamentous and muscular structure allow the body to perform extraordinary tasks as a result. Dancers are renowned for the extremes of their range of movement, much of which is effected through the hip and lumbo-pelvic region. It is well recognized that increases in range can reduce the inherent stability of any region in the body, but the impact in this particular region can be significant. Potential alterations to the bony morphology as a result of the training undertaken while bones are still developing, possibly in the case of femoral retroversion, can further alter the complex biomechanics of the lumbo-pelvic area. Furthermore, there may be an impact on any lower limb injury. Understanding these changes and challenges is key for any healthcare clinician working with dancers.

LUMBAR AND SACRAL REGION

Anatomy and Associated Pathology

As with all regions in the spine, the orientation of the facet joints determines the nature of the movement that occurs in that region. Within the lumbar region, the angle of the facets (up to 90 degrees in the lower lumbar region) allows for more movement into flexion and extension than rotation. Typically, there is increasing movement into flexion and extension lower down the lumbar region, with the lumbosacral region providing the greatest movement.

In dancers there can often be an alteration to this pattern, with greater movement into extension seen at the upper lumbar region, very limited range through the middle of the lumbar region and then excessive movement again in the lumbosac-

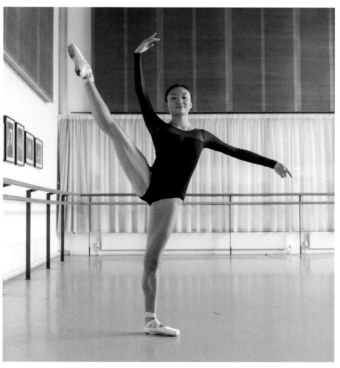

Photo 95   Dancer performing développé à la seconde.

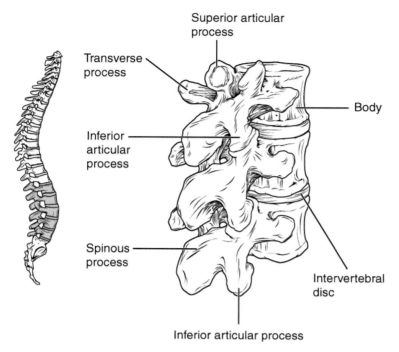

Superior articular process

Transverse process

Body

Inferior articular process

Spinous process

Intervertebral disc

Inferior articular process

Fig. 22   Bony anatomy of the lumbar region.

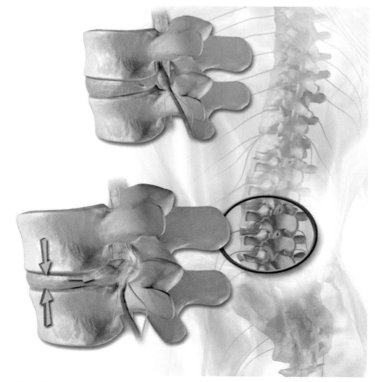

Fig. 23   Diagrammatic illustration of a lumbar disc protrusion.

ral region. This hinging in the upper lumbar region, along with a failure to control forces through the hypermobile segments, can cause it to become a site of injury, with reports of spondylolysis of the pars interarticularis (a bony column created between vertebrae) region. Although the prevalence of stress fractures is greater in female (ballet) dancers – potentially associated with a combination of greater ranges into extension used with challenges seen in REDs and female triad syndrome – there have been reports of male dancers sustaining bone stress injuries as well. The presence of spondylolisthesis has also been reported in dance. This change in normal mechanics needs careful monitoring and evaluation in the presence of lumbar symptoms. Unlike flexion and extension, the (limited) axial rotation and lateral flexion are shared equally through the various segments of the lumbar region.

The intervertebral discs serve to separate as well as connect the vertebral segments. The disc is comprised of central nucleus pulposes with the surrounding annulus fibrosus. The discs are joined with the hyaline cartilage end plates of the vertebral segments. There is a relatively lower prevalence of discogenic pathology in dance, with the majority of cases occurring in the lumbar region.

Although the problem may be seen in both genders, male dancers particularly have reported with acute herniation and sequestrated

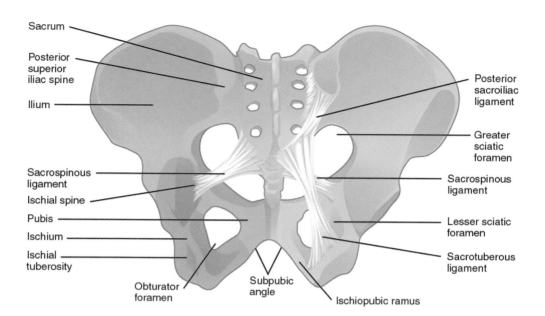

Fig. 24 Sacroiliac ligaments.

Sacrum
Posterior superior iliac spine
Ilium
Sacrospinous ligament
Ischial spine
Pubis
Ischium
Ischial tuberosity
Obturator foramen
Subpubic angle
Ischiopubic ramus
Posterior sacroiliac ligament
Greater sciatic foramen
Sacrospinous ligament
Lesser sciatic foramen
Sacrotuberous ligament

discs following lifts. A higher prevalence may reflect the nature of contemporary lifts, but contemporary ballet and ballroom have also seen biomechanically challenging lifts being performed. End-plate injuries, although not often reported in dance, need to be part of the overall differential diagnosis in low back pain considerations.

It is important when considering the biomechanics of the lumbar region to include the impact of its pelvic articulation. The impact of the sacroiliac joint can be underestimated in its role in contributing to trunk and lower limb movement. Moreover, because of the nature of dance, dancers will generally experience a greater transmission of ground forces up through the legs as opposed to axial loading. The role of the hips and sacroiliac joints in the conversion of torque is critical to the extent and nature of the load that is experienced in the lumbar region.

A simplistic model of load can show how ground reaction forces transmit loading through the legs upwards. This load is controlled/absorbed through the associated joints and muscles. In particular, the external rotation moment through the hips and the internal rotation moment through the sacroiliac joint greatly influence the resultant force experienced in the lumbar region (and beyond). Rehabilitation programmes can target control of the hips and

sacroiliac joint as a means to reduce loading through the lumbar region. The sacroiliac joint is made up of the sacrum, a triangular-shaped bone that sits between the iliac bones. Stability of the region is through a combination of form closure and force closure, essentially relating to static structures and dynamic stabilizers and their interaction, to provide a foundation of stability from which movement is supported. The static stabilizers include the bony architecture and ligamentous structures, including the sacrotubous ligament.

Tenderness on palpation of the sacrotubuous ligament can be a useful indicator of 'less than optimal stability' of the sacroiliac joint. Form closure is supported with the activation of key pelvic muscles. Mens et. al. developed a simple test for sacroiliac instability in post-partum women. The Mens test involves the patient lying supine and undertaking an active straight-leg raise to 5–15cm. A positive test is recorded if the patient experiences any pain or describes a difference in strength or ability of one leg compared with the other (often described as one leg feeling 'heavier' when lifted). For the purpose of interpretation, the pelvis can then be manually stabilized, providing force closure for the sacroiliac joint, and the test repeated to assess the impact of improving stability on the symptoms.

Movement of the sacrum (relative to the ilium) is described as nutation (flexion) and counternutation (extension). During hip flexion, the sacrum should nutate on the side of the flexed leg. During hip extension, the sacrum should counternutate on the side of the extended leg. During nutation, the long dorsal ligament is slack while during counternutation is becomes taut. The assessment of movement of the sacrum in hip flexion is a simple clinical tool to establish whether there is increased mobility (when compared with the opposite side) or blocked movement. Both create an important insight as to the stability of the region and the reactionary biomechanical changes that may be influencing symptoms or predisposition to injury. Assessment is done by the healthcare practitioner placing their left thumb on the patient's left posterior iliac spine and their right thumb on the sacrum. The patient is then instructed to raise their left knee to 90 degrees of hip flex. The movement of the ilium is then compared with right hip flexion in standing. Dysfunctional patterns may include a blocked or upward movement of the ilium.

Dynamic stabilizers of the sacroiliac joint include muscular slings. Key muscular slings for the sacroiliac joint include the longitudinal sling, posterior oblique sling and the anterior oblique sling. The longitudinal sling comprises the multifidus (attaching to the sacrum), thoracolumbar fascia and the long head of biceps and its attachment to the sacrotuberous ligament of the sacroiliac joint. The posterior oblique sling comprises the latissimus dorsi and gluteus maximus, while the anterior oblique

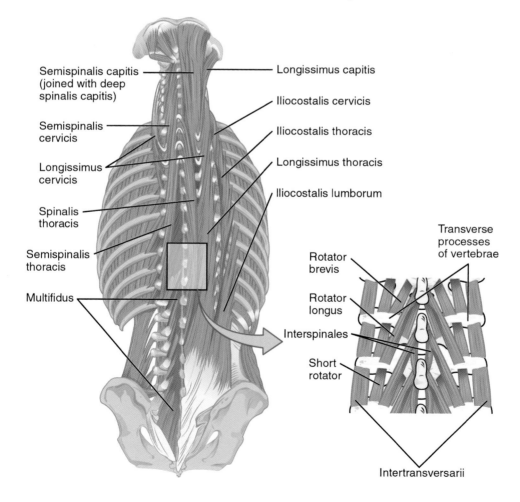

Semispinalis capitis (joined with deep spinalis capitis)

Semispinalis cervicis

Longissimus cervicis

Spinalis thoracis

Semispinalis thoracis

Multifidus

Longissimus capitis

Iliocostalis cervicis

Iliocostalis thoracis

Longissimus thoracis

Iliocostalis lumborum

Rotator brevis

Rotator longus

Interspinales

Short rotator

Transverse processes of vertebrae

Intertransversarii

**Fig. 25
Muscular anatomy of the spine.**

sling comprises the pectoralis, internal and external obliques and transverse abdominus.

Considering the multitude of structures and segments that contribute to the unique movement of the spine, it is unsurprising that the challenging condition of low back pain affects a large proportion of the general population. It is no different for sportspeople and dancers. The nature of dance can add specific stresses to the region. For the male dancer, there may be additional loading on to the lumbar region when lifting during partnering. Both genders in dance, and particularly ballet, are typically required to perform movements that entail (hyper-) extension at the lumbar spine. This is often combined with extension at the hip (in arabesque) for female dancers, who often push into extremes of range. In the younger or developing dancer, there is a risk of bone stress injury to the pars regions.

The load experienced in the lumbar region in jumping also plays a part in the increased prevalence of non-specific low back pain in dance. With many dance styles adopting a 'turn-out' position, an increased awareness needs to be placed on an assessment of the manner in which forces are transmitted up the kinetic chain, from the legs, through the hips and sacroiliac joint regions to the lumbar region. When undertaken correctly, turn-out occurs from the hips with the external rotators. The same muscles are also responsible for providing components of the dynamic stability of the lumbar sacral region, through the stabilization of the sacroiliac joints. Therefore, these are an important component of the conditioning and rehabilitation of dancers.

Rehabilitation of the Lumbo-Pelvic Region

When constructing a rehabilitation programme for the lumbar region it is important to consider the entire lumbo-pelvic complex and the forces affecting it (ground reaction and axial). This is particularly relevant in an assessment of how the sacroiliac region accepts the internal rotation moment and the hips accept the external moment. In addition to this, consideration should be given to the well-reported impact of the biopsychosocial factors that affect back pain.

Within the neuromuscular component of the rehabilitation, early stage focus would be on creating sacroiliac (and lumbar) stability. The post-partum active straight-leg test (Mens test) for sacroiliac joint instability is a useful starting point. The patient lies on their back, performs an active straight-leg raise to around 15cm, and identifies whether the exertion in lifting each leg is different or causes any discomfort or pain. This is then followed up with a manual stabilization of the pelvic cage, with the clinician placing compressive forces on the sacroiliac joint via the anterior, lateral or posterior pelvic cage. Reducing any reported 'heaviness' of a limb or pain demonstrates the influence of sacroiliac stability on mechanical loading through the lumbar pelvic region or pain provocation. Furthermore, it helps to establish the likely impact of form closure through force closure on symptoms or on the stability of the sacroiliac spine. It therefore helps establish the specific and tested starting point for the early-stage neuromuscular component of their rehabilitation or conditioning programme. The hip extensors and external rotators glut maximus and glut medius are also responsible for stabilization of the sacroiliac joint.

Isometric hip extension and external rotation exercises serve a dual purpose throughout the rehabilitation process. They will use the patient's own muscle work to provide improved stability through the sacroiliac joint. Due to the nature of reciprocal muscle activity, the activation of glut max may also serve to reduce the over-activation of the iliopsoas muscle group, which is often seen in a hypertonic protective response to low back pain in dancers. The implementation of neuromuscular programmes may also be used to address any movement competency issues that have been observed. The use of normal movement testing may help to identify areas where optimal movement patterning and control are not achieved.

An assessment of any strength deficit as part of an evaluation of the potential causes for lower back pain needs to include an assessment of the posterior chain. Although the role of 'typical' strength training, in the guise of Olympic lifting, is still an area of debate and discussion in dance, the role of the posterior chain and trunk extensors in lower back pain has been established and should be taken into account when planning a rehabilitation (and prevention) programme.

The functional integration component of the rehabilitation programme needs to look to address the functional activity that, through the history taking, may have been identified as a pain provocation, as well as areas that may contribute to the overall loading of the lumbar region. This might include lifting technique in male dancers. Here, an assessment of shoulder stability and range is needed, alongside the ability to maintain lumbar and thoracic curvature under load. If an assessment of jumping is warranted, then an evaluation of ankle range and control into dorsiflexion (both clinically and func-tionally) will help give an appreciation of the ability of the dancer to get their heels down in jumps, under control. The ability to do this makes a notable difference to the landing biomechanics and the subsequent forces that are transmitted up the chain.

Although it is much less prevalent, the pathology affecting the anterior aspect of the pelvis still needs to be considered. Lower abdominal strains, through the attachment of rectus abdominus, need to be explored and differentiated from other sources of hip and trunk flexion pathology, including iliopsoas and rectus femoris. Due to their origin on the pubic rami, the traction of the adductor group can cause both high signal changes on a T2 weighted MRI, suggesting bony involvement, as well as irritation of the pubic symphysis in osteitis pubis.

CASE STUDY 2: NON-SPECIFIC, MECHANICAL LOWER BACK PAIN

A male classical ballet dancer with an on-going history of lower lumbar pain following a lift. No red flags. A six-week rehabilitation programme was implemented to facilitate the functional requirements of lifting while supporting the lower back. In particular, emphasis was placed on developing aspects of the supporting muscular slings.

Table 9   Initial rehabilitation for lower lumbar pain.

Session 1 (2 weeks)	Time (sec)	Reps	Sets
Inhibition			
Foam roller releases	20–60		
Neuromuscular facilitation – isometric			
Isometric glute extension @ 90-deg hip flex	8	8	2
Isometric glute external rotation @ 90-deg hip flex	8	8	2
Sarhmann obliques	8	8	2
Sarhmann heel taps	8	8	2
Isolate/strengthen			
Concentric			
Swiss ball bridges		10	2
Swiss ball trunk prone extension		10	2
Eccentrics			
Swiss ball supine trunk rotations		10	2
Functional integration			
Plank – 3-point hold (alternate single limb lift)		8	2
Superman in 4-point kneeling	30	1	1

Table 10   Mid-stage rehabilitation programme for lower lumbar pain.

Session 2 (2 weeks)	Time (sec)	Reps	Sets
Inhibition			
Foam roller releases	20–60		
Neuromuscular facilitation – isometric			
Isometric glute extension @ 90-deg hip flex	8	8	2
Isometric glute external rotation @ 90-deg hip flex	8	8	2
Sarhmann obliques with heel lift	8	8	2
Sarhmann heel taps with heel slide	8	8	2
Isometric trunk holds (front, back, sides)	8	8	2
Isolate/strengthen			
Concentric			
Seated Swiss ball Arnold press		10	2
Side-lying hip internal and external rotation		10	2
Eccentrics			
Good mornings		10	2
Functional Integration			
Single-leg Romanian dead lift		8	2
Superman		8	2
Reach and pull		8	2

Table 11   End-stage rehabilitation programme for lower lumbar pain.

Session 3 (2 weeks)	Time (sec)	Reps	Sets
Inhibition			
Foam roller releases	20–60		
Neuromuscular facilitation – isometric			
Isometric trunk holds (front, back, sides)	20	2	1
Chariot pulls (front, back, sides)		8	2
Isolate/strengthen			
Concentric			
Bent over row		10	2
Side-lying hip internal and external rotation		10	2
Eccentrics			
Reverse incline pull-up		10	2
Functional integration			
Romanian dead lift		5	2
Water ball squat to shoulder press		8	2
Water ball press and step		8	2

HIP AND GROIN

Anatomy and Associated Pathology

The hip is a ball and socket joint that is comprised of the acetabulum of the pelvis with the head of the femur (ball). Through this, it achieves flexion and extension, abduction and adduction, and medial and lateral rotation. The acetabulum is a concave socket. Due to its shallow nature, it is deepened by a cartilaginous labrum, which increases the concavity of the acetabulum. The articulation is affected by various morphological variations. The position and depth of the acetabulum can vary, which can have an impact on both short- and long-term risk of injury, with potential secondary changes later in life. Similarly, within the femoral component, variations of the angle of inclination through the femoral neck can affect biomechanics and injury risk, not only to the hip, but also to the knee, sacroiliac joint and lower back.

Typically, when examining bone mineral density in dancers, it is seen to be lower in the lumbar region as opposed to the femoral neck, due to the weight-bearing nature of the activity. Despite this, femoral stress fractures can still be prevalent in dance. As part of the overall investigation, the potential presence of REDs needs to be explored, in particular the impact of amenorrhea with the lower energy availability. Typically, a stress fracture of the hip that occurs in the femoral neck is compression-based and can be treated without surgery. However, tension and displaced stress fractures are likely to require surgery, so an orthopaedic opinion will be required. Although rarely reported, the clinician should be aware of idiopathic osteoporosis of the hip when dealing with a dancer presenting with deep hip pain.

The angle of torsion of the femur can be to the front in femoral anteversion, or to the back in femoral retroversion. According to Hamilton et al., there

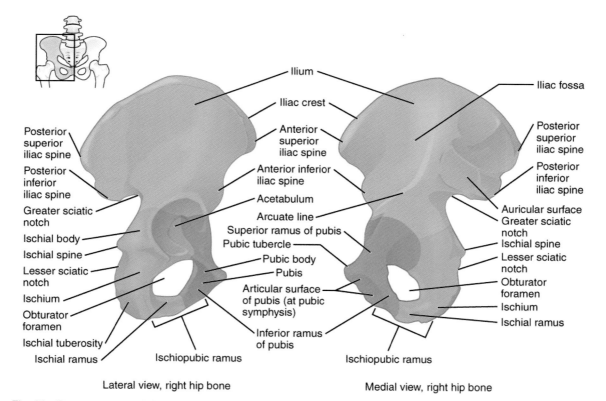

Lateral view, right hip bone   Medial view, right hip bone

Fig. 26   Bony anatomy of the hip joint.

is potentially a greater morphological retroversion variation seen in dancers. An assessment of this may form part of the talent identification process in younger age, as dancers with retroversion will appear to have greater turn-out from the hips. Its presence may, however, be a morphological adaptation due to the effects of the strain placed through the femur in training. Hamilton's work suggests that there is a relationship between intense classical dance training between 11 and 14 years of age and femoral retroversion. With femoral retroversion comes an increased risk of internal impingements of the labrum, so a greater understanding and evaluation are justified.

The joint is surrounded by a joint capsule and ligaments (iliofemoral, pubofemoral, ischiofemoral), providing a notable degree of the joint's stability. The stability of the hip is further enhanced by the twenty-two muscles that act upon it and consist of both deep and superficial layers. The major flexor of the hip is the iliopsoas, made up of psoas major, psoas minor and iliacus. Its origin at T12 to L5 and insertion at the lessor trochanter is important when considering a multitude of pain and pathology potentials with dancers. These can include its impact on the lumbar origin or the anterior hip joint and labrum.

Hip flexion is also assisted by the sartorius, rectus femoris and tensor fasica lata, so these need to be considered when looking at the impact of flexion-based pain and injury. There is a continuous relationship with the muscles of the hip and thigh with the tensor facia lata, which serves to improve efficiency of contractions around the hip by containing the muscles due to its inherent inelasticity. Snapping hip syndromes are not uncommon in dance. They can be internal or external. An internal snapping hip originates from the iliopsoas tendon snapping over the anterior hip joint. With an external snapping hip, the pain is experienced over the lateral hip due to the iliotibial band snapping over the trochanter. This can result in trochanteric

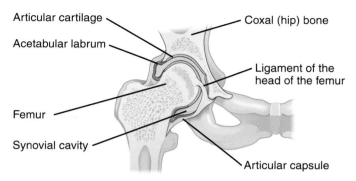

(a) Frontal section through the right hip joint

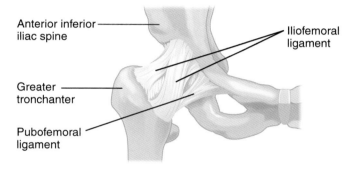

(b) Anterior view of right hip joint, capsule in place

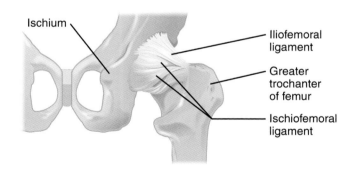

(c) Posterior view of right hip joint, capsule in place

Figs 27a–c   Anatomy and ligaments of the hip joint.

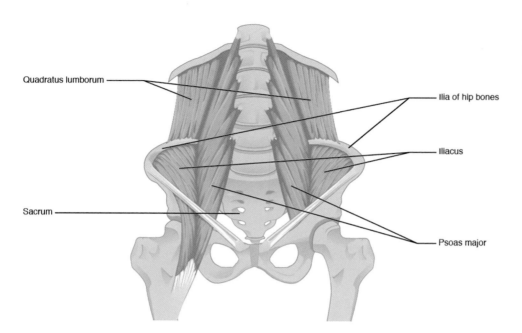

Quadratus lumborum

Sacrum

Ilia of hip bones

Iliacus

Psoas major

Fig. 28
Muscular
anatomy of the
anterior pelvis.

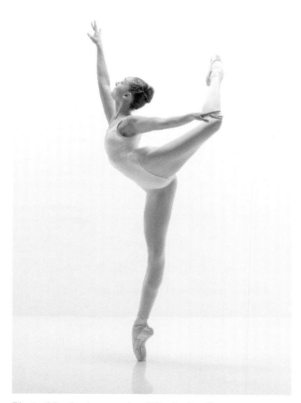

Photo 96   Arabesque in attitude derrière.
KIRSTY WALKER

bursitis, which can occur in dance when the bursa between the femur and iliotibial band rubs or is irritated. While it is important to exclude coexisting pathology from the hip joint, the greater trochanter is extra-capsular, so trochanteric bursitis will generally present in isolation, unlike iliopsoas bursitis, which has a strong correlation with labral pathology. Synovitis of the joint capsule is also a possibility, given the challenging forces that are put through this joint in dance.

The gluteus maximus is the key hip extensor. Often neglected, the adductor magnus is another key extensor when the hip is in flexion. Furthermore, with dancers it is important to recognize that hip extension can often be performed with lumbar extension, typically involving the upper lumbar region, in movements such as arabesque. The impact of this dual extension can result in compression of the lumbar region through the origin of psoas, or pressure on the anterior hip joint and labrum through the tension of the psoas tendon as it passes over towards its attachment to the lesser trochanter.

The role of the various hip muscles can vary depending on the position of the hip. Abduction is achieved via the gluteus medius and gluteus minimus when the hip is in extension, but they act

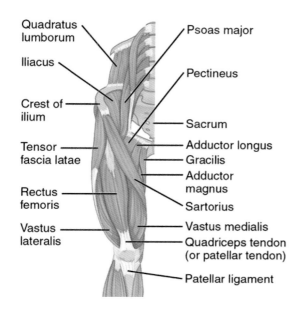

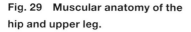

Fig. 29 Muscular anatomy of the
hip and upper leg.

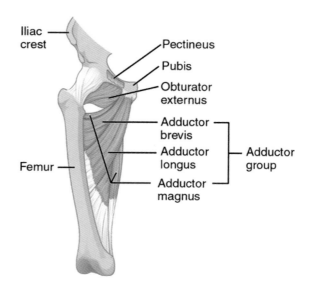

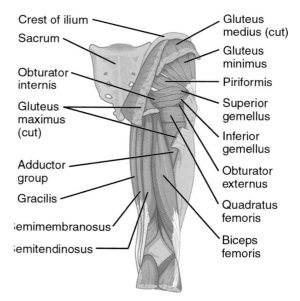

as internal rotators when the hip is flexed, along with tensor fascia lata. There are six primary lateral rotators, including piriformis, which also supports extension. The other rotators are the superior gemelli, obturator internus, obturator externus, inferior gemelli and quadratus femoris. Given the importance of turn-out from the hip in classical ballet, these form a significant part of examinations for both injury potential and their influence on biomechanics and subsequently through the kinetic chain. Hip adduction is achieved via the obturator externus and the adductor group that are attached to the pubic rami of the pelvis, comprised of the adductor magnus, adductor brevis, adductor longus, adductor minimus with pectineus, gracilis and obturator externus. Again, the angle of hip flexion is reflected in the dominant muscle activity, with the adductor magnus working between 0 and 60 degress, the adductor longus from 60 degrees and the pectineus at 90 degrees.

Given the nature of dance movements, in particular turn-out, optimum control through the hip is paramount. The hip adductors provide a counter lever to hip abduction. Within some sporting populations, adductor tendinopathy can be prevalent. In dance, adductor tendinopathy may be a result of an insufficiency of the adductor group for the loading (over time) or overloading as part of a compensatory activation to control a 'give' in abduction from the hip. Assessment of adductor region pain also includes a differential diagnosis of posterior abdominal wall disruptions, where small tears in the oblique muscles are noted in the vicinity of the inguinal ligament/femoral triangle. These need to be evaluated against potential compression of the femoral genital nerve, which will refer pain to the inguinal region without the structural compromise seen with tears of the oblique muscle wall. It is important in this region not to miss a stress response (or fracture) of the femoral neck. Management of a femoral neck bony stress injury requires immediate offloading. An understanding of potential bone stress risks, including vitamin D status, bone mineral density and menstrual status (in females) is important.

Management of adductor tendinopathy in dancers comprises a focus on eccentric loading of the adductor, alongside improved control of the hip abduction and external rotation. A similar programme can be used for the longer-term management of osteitis pubis.

Impingement Symptoms

Given the reported increased prevalence of acetab-ular retroversion, acetabular dysplasia and femoral retroversion in dancers in comparison with the general population, femoral acetabular impingement (FAI) is clearly an important consideration. It is more prevalent in ballet dancers. As in sporting populations, this impingement can be due to cam or pincer, or mixed, presentations. A further consideration is the presence of an os acetabuli. Like the os trigonum in the posterior aspect of the ankle, this may provide a source of bony impingement in the hip. The impact of the impingement potential due to bony changes can result in damage to the acetabular labrum. As part of the examination of a potential labral tear it is important to exclude a differential diagnosis of posterior pelvic pain. Patients with posterior pelvic pain may present with pain and/or heaviness during the Mens active straight-leg test. More importantly, they report posterior pain when performing a hip compression test. With labral tears, patients will often present with a 'C' sign – indicating their hip pain using a 'C' shape with their hand. It is important to match history, presenting symptoms and clinical findings with results of radiology (in this instance, a magnetic resonance arthrogram, or MRA). As with a shoulder labral tear, standard

Table 12   Adductor tendinopathy rehabilitation session.

Tendinopathy session	Time (sec)	Reps	Sets
Inhibition			
Foam roller releases – quads, hams and gluts	20–60		
Neuromuscular facilitation – isometric			
Glut med/max isometric holds in side-lying and hip flex and external rotation	8	8	2
Isometric adductor holds at 0, 60, 90deg	45–60	4	2
Isolate/strengthen			
Eccentrics			
Side-lying adductor 'controlled drops' with load	NA	15	3
Controlled eccentric squats with adductor squeeze	NA	15	3
Functional integration			
Side plank lowering		12–15	3–4
Ski fitter lateral slides		12–15/ direction	3–4
Monster walks with emphasis on push-off leg		12–15/ direction	3–4

**Photo 97   Rosie Kay
Dance Company.**
BRIAN SLATER

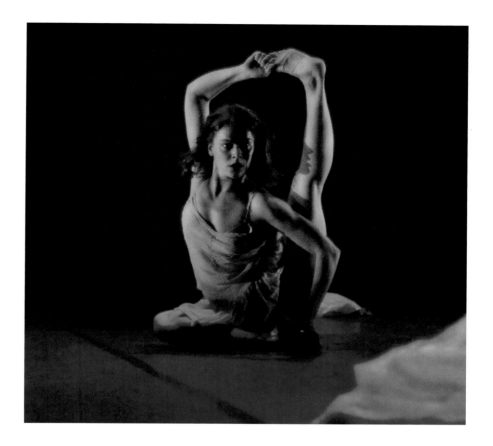

MRI may be insufficient to identify damage in the hip. Not all labral tears require surgical intervention and a full assessment of the influencing factors (intrinsic and extrinsic) is needed to determine the correct care pathway. This may range from nonsteroidal anti-inflammatory drugs (NSAIDs) with rehabilitation exercises, via guided steroid injections all the way to surgery.

While bony morphology can play a key role in the prevalence of these conditions, muscle balance and optimal biomechanics, due to the extreme range required in a dancer's hips, are paramount.

Assessment of the stability of the sacroiliac joint is an important part of the overall evaluation. There is a strong clinical correlation between the compensatory over-active iliopsoas muscle tone and decreased stability in the sacroiliac joint. An over-active psoas muscle can have a negative impact on hip movements and increase the

prevalence of impingement symptoms, particularly through extension and elevation through abduction, or arabesque and à la seconde, in dancing terms. This is a complex region, with the interactions of multiple muscles pulling around the pelvic cage. Assessment in a dancer needs to incorporate the pubic symphysis as a region that takes the strain, with the various stresses placed through the anterior pelvis.

The rehabilitation programme detailed in Case Study 3 was based on a 9-month period, extending beyond the 4- to 6-month period that might be expected with this type of surgery. The decision to extend it was made to allow a number of key criteria to be achieved. The acetabular tear was present in the absence of notable or clinically significant bony morphological changes, such as cam or pincer impingement signs, or a traumatic onset/inciting event as a mechanism. As a result, the healthcare

CASE STUDY 3: FEMORAL ACETABULAR IMPINGEMENT (FAI) IN DANCE

A male ballet dancer with a history of femoral acetabular impingement. The acetabular labrum was repaired surgically.

Table 13   Rehabilitation programme for a superior labral tear.

WEEK	1	2	3–4	5–8	9–12	13–16	17+
Phase 1 – protect and prepare (for loading)							
Range of movement (CPM 10deg to 90deg) (every 2 hours)	•						
Range of movement (CPM 7deg to 115deg) (every 2 hours)		•					
Active range of movement – ankle dorsiflexion and plantar flexion (every hour)	•	•					
Active range of movement – hip flexion – heels slides (every 2 hours)	•	•					
Active range of movement – hip rotation – controlled bent-knee fall-outs (every 2 hours)	•	•					
Gait re-education – focus on heel toe and good pelvic alignment	•	•					
Core session 1 (daily)	•	•					
Static bike (daily)		•	•	•	•	•	•
Phase 2 – ROM/core/proprioception							
Balance session (BIODEX, AIRex mat, BOSU ball) (2 × day)		•	•				
Preparation for strength session (daily)		•	•	•			
Pool/ hydrotherapy work (post suture removal at 2 weeks if wounds are clean and healed) (daily)			•	•			
Core session 2 (daily)			•	•			
Phase 3 – Functional strength and power							
Strength session 1 (3 × week)					•		
Power session 1 (3 × week)						•	•
Strength session 2 (3 × week)						•	•
Technical coaching (daily)					•	•	
Phase 4 – Functional Integration							
Class						•	
Rehearsal							•
Performance							•

Table 14   Core exercises.

	Reps	Sets	Rest
Core session 1			
Abductor isometric squeeze (0/45/90deg)	3x6–10sec hold/range	3	6–10sec
Sharman obliques	7–12	3	30sec
Sharman heel taps (within range of hip)	8–12	3	30sec
Isometric short clams @ 30-deg hip flex (with resistance band)	8–12	3	30sec
Isometric long clams @ 10-deg hip ext (with ankle weight if req.)	8–12	3	30sec
Prone hip extension (iso hold end range for 5 secs)	8–12	3	30sec
Bent-knee fall-out	8–12	3	30sec

Table 15   Strength exercises preparation.

	Reps	Sets	Rest
Preparation for strength session			
Resistance band ankle push and pull through	15–25	4	30sec
4-point kneeling superman holds (diagonals 10sec hold)	8–12	3	30sec
Plank	3–5 ×30sec hold	3	30sec
Lateral Plank	3–5 ×30sec hold	3	30sec
Isometric hip thruster with load	3–5 ×30sec hold	3	30sec
Reverse glut/hamstring raise	8–12	3	30sec

Table 16   Further core exercises.

	Reps	Sets	Rest
Core session 2			
Swiss ball prone/supine lateral roll-outs	8–12/position	2	30sec
Swiss ball plank with single-leg lifts	7–12	3	30sec
Swiss ball bridge	8–12	3	30sec
Swiss ball jack knife	8–12	3	30sec
Swiss ball hamstring pulls	9–12	3	30sec
Swiss ball sprinter's drill	8–12	3	30sec

(continued overleaf)

CASE STUDY 3: FEMORAL ACETABULAR IMPINGEMENT (FAI) IN DANCE *(continued)*

Table 17   Strength exercises.

	Reps	Sets	Rest
Strength session 1			
Reformer squats	15–25	4	30sec
Reformer plié to rise	15–25	4	30sec
Loaded hip extension/thrusts	3–6	4–6	30sec
Loaded side-lying hip internal rotation (hip 90deg)	3–6	4–6	30sec
Loaded side-lying hip external rotation (hip 90deg)	3–6	4–6	30sec
Body weight squats	8–12	4–6	30sec
Body weight lateral squats	8–12	4–6	30sec

Table 18   Power exercises.

	Reps	Sets	Rest
Power session 1			
Pogos	30sec	1	30sec
Hop and hold (front and back)	6–8	1	30sec
Hop and hold (lateral)	6–8	1	30sec
Squat jumps	6–8	1	30sec
Lateral squat rebound jumps	6–8	1	30sec
Split squat jumps	6–8	1	30sec
Jump box explosive jumps (2 leg to 2 legs)	6–8	1	1 min
Jump box explosive jumps (2 leg to 1 leg)	6–8	1	1 min
Jump box explosive jumps (1 leg to 2 legs)	6–8	1	1 min
Jump box explosive jumps (1 leg to 1 legs)	6–8	1	1 min
Jump box controlled landing (2 legs to 2 legs)	6–8	1	1 min
Jump box controlled landing (2 legs to 1 leg)	6–8	1	1 min

Table 19   Further strength exercises.

	Reps	Sets	Rest
Strength session (p.m.)			
Romanian dead lift	3–6	5	1min
Front squats	3–6	5	1min
Loaded hip extension/thrusts	3–6	5	1min
Sumo squats	3–6	5	1min
Lateral squat	3–6	5	1min
Turkish get up	8–12	3	1min

clinician automatically suspected biomechanical or technical anomalies. An extended rehabilitation period was designed to allow the key phases to be longer, in particular the strength and technical phase. When technical changes are established, it is important to implement supportive exercise programmes to facilitate those changes, as well as to give time for the required strength and/or power changes to be consolidated.

The specific exercises are given in Tables 14-18.

While dancers are accustomed to establishing quick movement pattern changes, having a highly skilled approach to learning new choreography, this does not equate to strength changes. They need a reasonable amount of time to consolidate strength changes physiologically as part of the rehabilitation design and timeline. Implementing a 'true' strength programme in dance can also be a challenge, especially in the face of concerns about hypertrophy. The principle of 'time under load', using blood flow restriction training as opposed to overload, is sometimes useful to bridge that gap. This may involve a series of targeted exercises using one set of 30 repetitions followed by three sets of 15 repetitions at around 20 per cent of the 1RM.

Following a successful return to full dance, a maintenance programme can be employed to maintain the correct control of optimal biomechanics. The components are typically selected from key findings from the assessment. Table 20 is an example of the maintenance programme employed for the surgical case described in Case Study 3.

Table 20   Maintenance programme following successful hip surgery.

Exercise and progression	Progressive overload		
	Reps per set	Sets	Rest between sets
1. Side-lying isometric hip extension			
	3–5/leg with 7-sec hold	2	3 secs between contract
2. Side-lying isometric hip ext rotation	3–5/leg with 7-sec hold	2	3 secs between contract
3. Swiss ball straight-leg bridge (SL)	6–8	2	30sec
4. Swiss ball reverse bridge (SL)	6–8	2	30sec
5. Swiss ball hamstring pulls	6–8	2	30sec
3. Side-lying leg lift (int rot)	6–8	3	30sec
4. Side-lying leg lift (ext rot)	6–8	3	30sec
5. 3-point heel lifts with resistance band	6–8	3	30sec
7. Monster resistance band walks	10/direction	2–4	30sec
8. Lunge walks or standing scooter	8–10	2	30sec

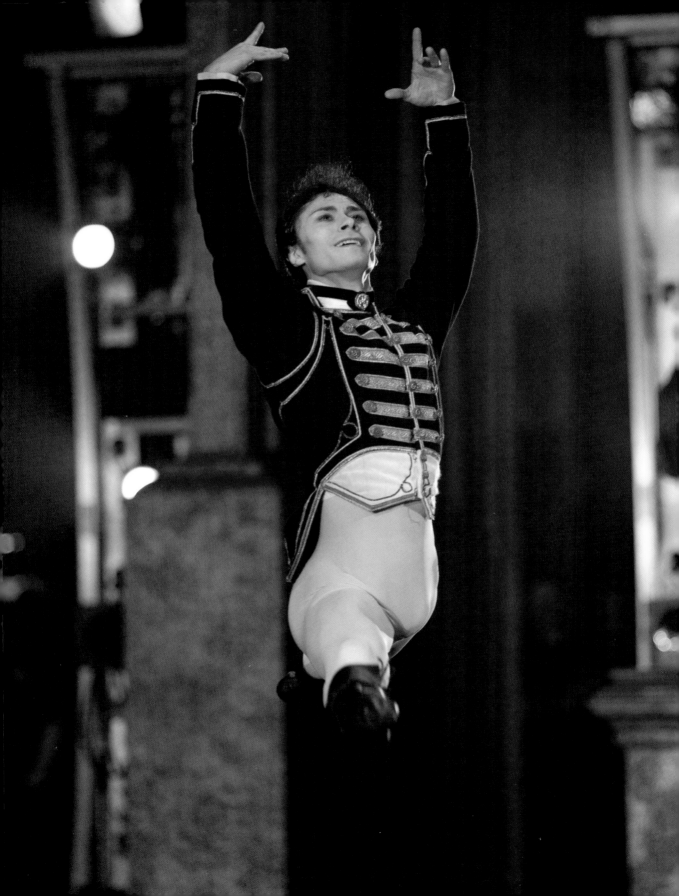

CHAPTER 9

UPPER LEG AND KNEE INJURIES

Much of the story-telling in dance derives from the control and power that dancers are able to produce. There is a significant impact on the upper leg and knee, and this area is therefore a key issue for consideration in dance. As in most sports, the knee is vulnerable to traumatic and impact injuries as a result of jumps or slips, as well as overuse injuries through repeated loading. The research literature suggests that major injuries of the knee, such as anterior cruciate ligament (ACL) disruptions, can lead to an increased risk of developing secondary changes such as osteoarthritis. It is therefore important for an attending clinician to be aware of the impact of returning dancers from these injuries before full rehabilitation has been achieved. This chapter will review the anatomy of the upper leg and knee and discuss the type of injuries that dancers may sustain, as well as offer potential rehabilitation plans as part of an overall management programme.

UPPER LEG

Anatomy and Related Pathology

Like the lower leg, the upper leg comprises a number of compartments. There are three – the anterior, medial and posterior – separated, as in the lower leg, by the intermuscular septum. The anterior compartment contains the muscle groups responsible for the extension of the knee: the quadriceps (vastus medialis, vastus lateralis, vastus intermedialis and rectus femoris) and sartorius. The insertion of the iliopsoas group also sits within the anterior compartment. The role of the psoas as a hip flexor is well understood. The angle of activation is generally assumed to be around 90 degrees of hip flexion,

but this can vary significantly. Hip flexor strains and tears can be prevalent in dance, and it is important to identify the source of such injury as part of a diagnosis and management strategy. It may have originated in either the iliopsoas or the rectus femoris, both of which sit in the anterior compartment.

The medial compartment contains the adductor group of muscles, which originate on the pubic bones. The lumbar pelvic anatomy comprises the pubic symphysis, and the nature of dance movements, and the traction of the adductors on the pubic rami, leads to the possibility of osteitis pubis. Certain choreography and movements in dance can result in an overloading of the adductor group and as such increase the potential for overuse injuries, both to the tendinous sections and to their origins in the pubic rami. Furthermore, much of dance requires good stabilization from the external rotators and abductors of the hip. A lack of stability in this movement of the hip – in other words, if there is a lateral 'give' in the hip – can result in compensatory over-activity of the adductors as part of a dysfunctional attempt to stablish and control movements of the hip (see Chapter 8).

The posterior compartment houses the flexor group of muscles. These muscles work to extend the hip and flex the knee. The impact of the sciatic nerve here is important. The sciatic nerve exits the hip through the sciatic foramina, beneath the piriformis muscle. Increased tone of the piriformis or the gemellus muscle can cause pressure on the sciatic nerve, causing an intermittent peripheral nerve entrapment, sometimes called piriformis syndrome. The significance of such an entrapment is the absence of nerve damage or pathology, but

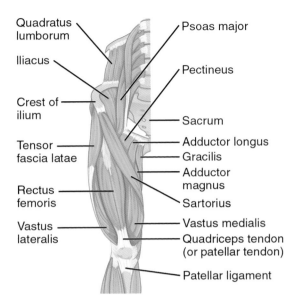

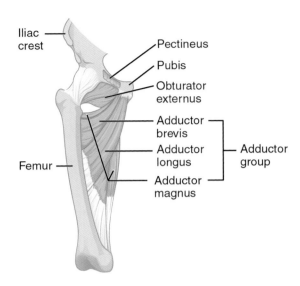

Fig. 30   Muscular anatomy of the upper leg and hip.

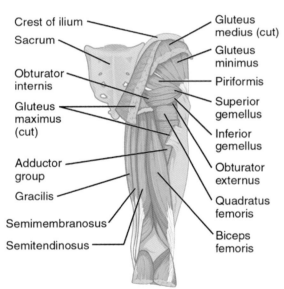

the presence of inflammation. Critically, intermittent nerve entrapments are also reversible.

Due to the excessive workload of the external rotators of the hip in dancers, a potential for these presentations exists and therefore the attending healthcare practitioner needs to be aware and testing for their presence. The origins of the hamstring group to the ischial tuberosity and sacral region is an important factor of the posterior compartment. Hypertonic changes seen in the bicep group as a result of less than optimal stability of the sacroiliac joint, through the identification of a loss of hamstring elongation/length, is a key clue to establishing the presence of the sacroiliac joint as part of the injury differentiation in this region. The biceps femoris insertion into the head of the fibula is also an important consideration when exploring the potential dysfunctional biomechanics in the presence of overuse injuries. Biceps femoris, through its origin and insertion, has the capacity to externally rotate the hip as well as the leg (from the knee). With a large part of ballet performed in a turned-out position, the role of biceps femoris is often underestimated. The medial hamstrings, semimembranosus and semitendinosus, are also fundamental in dance, playing a vital role in knee flexion, particularly in flexing the knee in à la seconde.

These issues become important when making decisions about tendon replacements for anterior cruciate ligament reconstructions, where the semimembranosus is often a ligament of choice. While

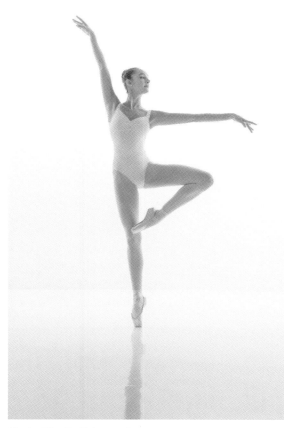

Photo 98 Retiré passé. KIRSTY WALKER

this hamstring plays a role in dance-specific movements, this does not mean it should be excluded from considerations for grafts – just that extra care needs to be taken within the rehabilitation programme to ensure the movement is restored post-surgery.

Muscle Injuries of the Upper Leg

The prevalence of upper-leg muscle tears or strains through hamstring and quadricep groups is low in comparison with some sporting populations. The nature of movement in dance may lead to more problems with the quadriceps than with the hamstrings. As there is a clear relationship to lower back pain, as well as anterior cruciate ligament injury, lower-leg conditioning programmes for dancers should include a balanced approach to posterior chain muscle work, including the hamstrings.

Like the later system developed by British Athletics, the classification system detailed in the 2012 Munich Consensus Statement gives the attending clinician a more specific means by which to describe and document the nature of muscle pathology. It does however still rely on the use of radiological support, which may not always be available. While imaging is useful in giving an accurate

THE MUNICH CONSENSUS STATEMENT ON MUSCLE INJURY

There are various grading systems relating to muscle injury, but in 2012 the Munich Consensus Statement on muscle injuries in sport set out to clarify and agree the terminology of the classification of such injuries. The statement offered a new classification system, which differentiated between four types of functional muscle disorders:

- **Type 1:** overexertion-related
- **Type 2:** neuromuscular muscle disorders
  (Both are used to describe disorders without macroscopic evidence of fibre tear and structural muscle injuries.)
- **Type 3:** partial tears
- **Type 4:** (sub-) total tears/tendinous avulsions) with macroscopic evidence of fibre tear/structural damage

The statement went on to offer subclassifications of each type as well.

description of the injury and extended evidence, to help establish potential timelines for return to dance, a well-structured rehabilitation programme can still be followed without it. The use of the incremental loading of targeted muscle groups seen in accelerated muscle rehabilitation programmes (notably in hamstring rehabilitation) can be undertaken, as long as the patient is carefully cued to respect the threshold of pain. The premise behind the accelerated rehab programme is based on early mobilization and strengthening of damaged fibres, without extending the lesion further. Giving clear instructions to stay below the threshold of pain and careful monitoring will ensure that this is possible.

An adapted acceleration programme for the quad can be implemented on a Pilates reformer. The patient is supine on the reformer with a low resistance level set through the spring system. They perform 3 sets of increasing reps at the low level of resistance (1 x 10 reps, 1 x 20 reps, 1 x 30 reps) with a 30-second recovery between sets. They then rest for 1 minute and then repeat, with an increased resistance through the spring system. This is continued with increasing resistance until an awareness of symptoms or fatigue is reported. The patient is then put through an active recovery process, including a 'warm-down' at low resistance, stretching, compression and possibly ice if the muscle is a little uncomfortable. The session is repeated daily, starting from the beginning again (with low resistance). Once a suitable level is achieved, the programme is taken into a weightbearing position (for example, squats). Again, as a suitable level of resistance is tolerated, additional aspects of function are included, including more plyometric aspects.

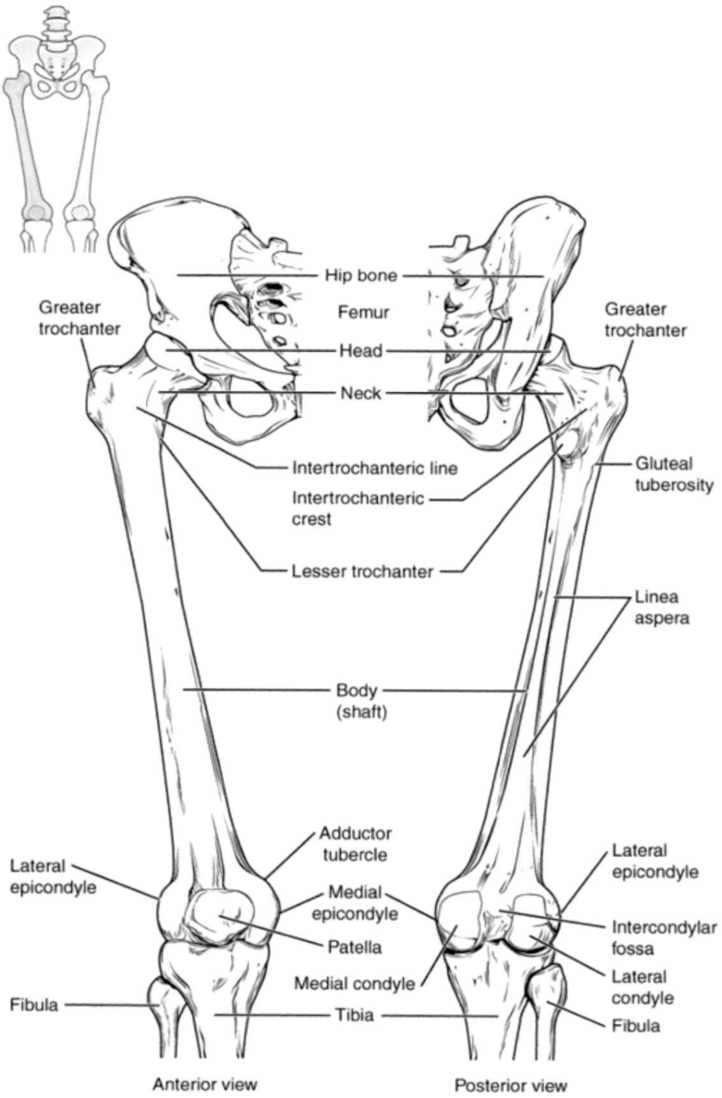

KNEE

Anatomy and Related Pathology

The knee is a complex joint, comprising the femur, tibia and patella. It is considered to be both a hinge and pivot joint, offering rotation and translatory movement.

An expected range of flexion in the knee is from -5 to around 160 degrees. With the higher prevalence of hypermobility in dancers, hyper-

Fig. 31   Bony anatomy of the upper leg and knee.

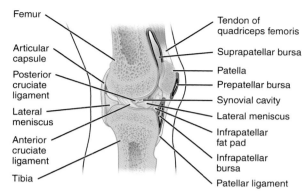

(a) Sagittal section through the right knee joint

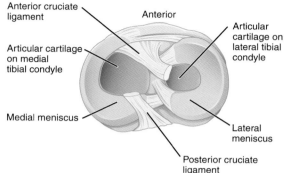

(b) Superior view of the right tibia in the knee joint, showing the menisci and cruciate ligaments

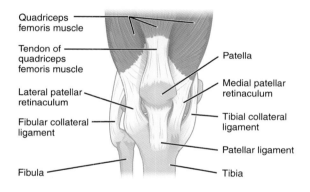

(c) Anterior view of right knee

Figs 32a–c   Anatomy of the knee joint, including meniscus and anterior muscles.

extension of the knee is not unusual. (Using the Beighton score criteria, a flexion of greater than -10 degrees would indicate hypermobility.) Around 25 degrees of rotation is seen through the knee in a flexed position. Turn-out is an important aspect of classical ballet, which should be done from the hip. However, dancers will sometimes turn out from the lower leg through the knee instead. This should be avoided. Continuous and excessive turn-out from the knee may result in laxity and increase the risk of instability and subsequent injury, potentially to the meniscal and articular cartilage.

From extension to flexion, the femoral condyle will roll in the first 25 degrees and then roll and glide. According to Masouros and fellow authors, the anterior cruciate ligament plays a vital role in preventing the further movement of the femur. The ACL also plays a role in providing rotation stabil-

ity, restricting excessive pivoting through the knee. The knee is supported by a further three major ligaments, including the posterior cruciate ligament, which restricts movement of the tibia posteriorly to the femur. Medial and lateral collateral ligaments provide stability against valgus and varus stresses. Additionally, there is support from the medial retinaculum, including the patellofemoral ligament and lateral retinaculum, quadriceps and patella tendons. Furthermore, the medial aspect is support through the presence of semimembranosus and laterally with bicep femoris. There is also some suggestion that the gastrocnemius provides some dynamic stability of the posterior knee.

Extension of the knee is achieved through the respective angle pulls of the quadricep muscle groups. The role of the patella is to increase the lever length of the thigh and increase forces through the quadriceps. It is subject to numerous forces through its various soft-tissue attachments (lateral retinaculum, vastus lateralis and the iliotibial tract, medial retinaculum, vastus medialis, quadricep tendon and patella tendon). Variations on the 'Q' angle also

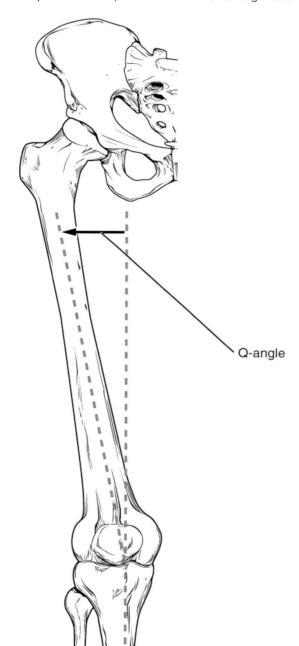

Q-angle

Fig. 33 'Q' angle in a female.

have an impact on the amount of force experienced through the patella. (The 'Q' angle is the angle created at the intersection of two imaginary lines, one drawn through the patella to the anterior superior iliac spine and the other drawn from the tibial tubercle through the patella; it is greater in females because they have a wider pelvis.)

The patella tendon is known to present with pathological adaptation due to the nature of the forces through the region. The compressive forces seen through the patella increase as knee flexion increases. This has been shown to result in potential impingement of Hoffa's fat pad as well as causing damage to the retro patella and femoral articular cartilage regions. The inelasticity seen with patella tendinopathy may have an impact on the increased patella compressive force and as such needs to be considered in both the management of chondral damage and in looking at preventive and long-term plans. An asymmetrical amount of lateral force on the patella due to insufficient pull of the medial structures has been associated with (lateral) maltracking of the patella, which can also lead to impingement of the fat pad and articular damage to femoral and patella chondral surfaces.

As the femoral condyles are rounded and the corresponding tibia is flattened, the knee joint relies on the medial and lateral menisci for stability and to assist with load-bearing. The role of the meniscus in load distribution is important when considering management of injuries that include this zone and its potential to heal. The posterior knee includes the popliteal fossa with the popliteal muscle and tendon, which play an important role in stabilizing tibial torsion and may be strained when dancers are forcing their turn-out from the lower leg as opposed to the hip, which is the desired action.

Soft-Tissue Injuries of the Knee

While most injuries to the knee are noted in the anterior aspect, it is important to consider the posterior knee when dancers present with knee pain. The presence of a Baker's cyst may be a strong indicator of an underlying meniscal tear. The role of the popliteus in controlling tibial rotation also needs to be considered in dancers with knee pain. Dancers who force their turn-out from their lower leg as opposed to the hip may experience pain from the popliteal muscle or adaptive changes to the popliteal tendon. Assessment of tibial rotation in sitting (90 degrees of knee flexion) can allow some appreciation of the strain through the knee. Comparison with the unaffected knee is important. If over-rotation is noted, an assessment of the control of tibial rotation is required. This can be performed in the same sitting position. The tibia is passively externally rotated. The clinician places their hand on the medial border of the foot and the patient is instructed to internally rotate their lower leg back to neutral. The clinician can assess the power and control that the patient has. They should also be looking for evidence of compensatory activation – typically, this might involve an over-active tibialis posterior, with the foot being inverted as part of the movement, as opposed to a neutral talocrural position being maintained as the tibia returns to neutral.

Patella Tendinosis and Hoffa's Fat Pad Impingements

The term 'patellofemoral pain syndrome' (PFPS) is used to describe pain experienced in the anterior aspect of the knee. It may originate from a variety of sources, and it is important to differentiate the location and causation of such pain if a management plan is to be successful. The physiological requirements of dance lead to a significant reporting of overuse injuries, including adaptive tendinosis changes in the patella tendons. These may occur in isolation in conjunction with Hoffa's fat pad impingement. It is important to differentiate between the origins of symptoms, as management of a fat pad impingement will involve a period of relative offload and inflammatory control, while tendon changes will benefit from a loading programme. Both will also require an evaluation of biomechanics as part of the understanding of causation.

It is an area of continued evolving thought, but the combination of tendon stripping injections under ultrasound guidance and an eccentric loading programme has yielded successful results in dancers. Further support of the tendon can be achieved through the supplementation of Vitamin D (very low levels of which have been recorded in dancers) and Omega 3. The impact of lateral patella maltracking needs to be taken into account in the rehabilitation process. Isometric contractions (45–60 second holds) can help with pain management. Nonsteroidal anti-inflammatories for up to a month have been advocated for fat pad impingements, prior to considering an ultrasound-guided steroid injection, if there is deemed to be a risk of fat pad atrophy. Dry needling of the diseased tendon can also be used to promote healing of the tendon. This may be done with the addition of platelet-rich plasma (PRP).

Given the functional requirements of the tendon in jumping in dance, and the amount of force experienced in it, heavy loading is recommended when implementing a loading programme. This will not only improve the tendon's tensile loading capacity, but also help condition the thigh muscles that play a key role in absorbing the remarkable forces that are felt during landing from jumps. A typical loading programme will start with isometric holds of 45–60 seconds (with a straight leg, if bent is not tolerated), up to four times a day. Eccentric loading is undertaken daily. The programme is based around single-leg eccentric squats using a 25-degree wedge squat board. Supported by Mark Youngs' research findings in 2005 for jumping athletes continuing to train and play with patella tendinopathy pain, this entails three sets of 15 repetitions twice a day. When the load is well tolerated, additional load can be applied.

The influence of an over-active tensor fascia latae (TFL) is considered one of the possible risk factors for developing patella tendinopathy. This over-activity may be associated with under-activity of the medial quadriceps as well as a biomechanical failure to control lateral glide and rotation of the hip. Additional exercises should be included to address this. The forces experienced by the tendon during jumping far outweigh those experienced during heavy slow strength-based exercising. Therefore, while it is safe and a useful means to increase load as part of the rehabilitation programme, it is important to develop both power and power endurance as part of a return to dance, and in particular

Table 21   Patella tendinopathy rehabilitation session.

Tendinopathy session	Time (sec)	Reps	Sets
Inhibition			
Foam roller releases – quads, hams and gluts	20–60		
Neuromuscular facilitation – isometric			
Glut med/max isometric holds in flex and ext	8	8	2
Isometric knee extension or if tolerated flexion	45–60	4	2
Isolate/strengthen			
Eccentrics			
25-deg eccentric squats (twice daily)	NA	15	3
Hip eccentric external rotations	NA	15	3
Functional integration			
Hop and holds on to 1 leg (controlled landing through foot/knee/hip)		12–15	3–4
Jump box landing drill (controlled landing through foot/knee/hip)		12–15	3–4
Jump box take offs drill (controlled landing through foot/knee/hip)		12–15	3–4

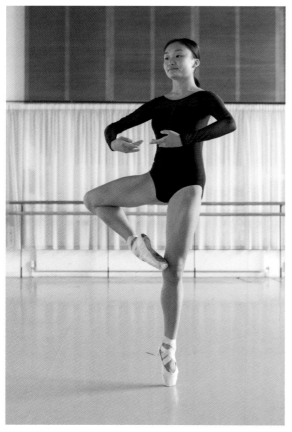

Photo 99   Dancer performing à passé.

to jumping. Finally, there is the ability to influence the mechanics that operate through the lower limb during landing. This entails an assessment of the dancer's ability to land effectively through their foot, followed by absorbing the forces through the knee and hip (under control).

The Victorian Institute of Sport Assessment (Patella) or VISA-P tool is useful to assess the fluctuations and patterns of symptoms associated with patella tendinopathy.

Bursitis

Soft-tissue irritation of the insertional region of the iliotibial band and the associated bursa is possible in dancers, with tightness of the band noted where there is insufficient control from the hip. Similar to ITB (iliotibial band) syndrome, on the medial aspect, is the increased risk of pes ans bursitis or tendon overload. Dancers, through the use of passé movements, can find themselves overloading the medial hamstring and the pes ans tendons.

Following a period to settle local inflammatory markers in the case of bursitis, management involves the development of pelvic stability alongside a tendon-loading programme following a typical tendinopathy strategy.

When performing some of the ground work associated with contemporary dance and some balletic choreographies, dancers can be at risk of sustaining traumatic pre-patella bursitis. Knee pads may not be allowed during performances, but their use during rehearsal will reduce the load through the knee. Given the proximity to the patella tendon, any decision to inject needs to be carefully evaluated, including a full appreciation of patella tendon health.

Ligament Injuries
Although the prevalence of ligament rupture around the knee is low in dancers, due to the potential severity and impact, it is an area that requires attention. Damage to the medial collateral ligament (MCL) is less frequent. Patients may report following trauma resulting from an awkward jump or lift.

With the deep fibres of the MCL being intracapsular, patients may present with some intracapsular swelling. Management of an intact MCL injury may involve a short period of immobilization of the ligament, to encourage it to reduce to its normal length, but maintenance of muscle mass and range of movement remains important in this period. Activation of the medial quadriceps as well as eccentric control of the external hip rotators form a fundamental part of the rehabilitation process. Damage to the lateral collateral ligament is less frequent due to the nature of the movement, coupled with the extensive soft-tissue support in the region. While the prevalence is very low, the mechanism seen in ACL disruptions with an extended knee may result in further tissue disruption, including the posterior lateral corner, consisting of the lateral collateral liga-

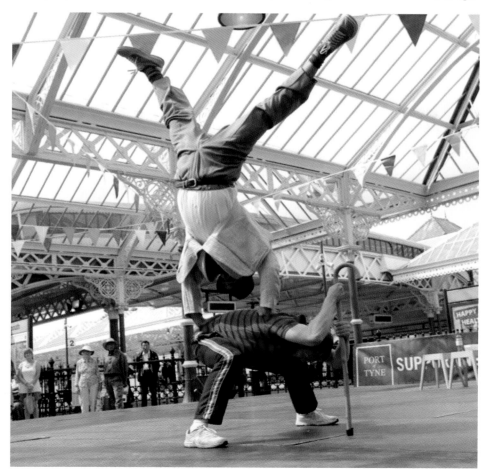

Photo 100 Challenging lifting while performing for 2FacedDance Company

ment, popliteal fibular ligament, iliotibial band, bicep femoris and lateral retinaculum. The injury may include damage to the anterior or posterior cruciate ligament. Some researchers have indicated that the time to diagnose a posterior lateral corner injury can be up to 8 months; it is often missed in the presence of more prevalent injuries such as ACLs. The 'dial' test should be performed in any serious knee injury, to avoid this, as radiology in the early stages may not always indicate damage to this area.

Anterior Cruciate Ligament Injuries

As in all sports, an anterior cruciate ligament injury has important implications in dance. The prevalence of concomitant meniscal and medial collateral ligament injury has been noted. The mechanism for injury has included both take-off for and landing from jumps. An ACL disruption can result in damage to the articular surface, creating a chondral defect.

Surgical opinion relating to the choice of graft needs to be taken into account. One of the key areas for inclusion in the decision-making is the dancer's functional need, which includes the ability to kneel and jump. Traditionally, the choice has been to use hamstring-based grafts, but the introduction of allografts may eliminate the complications. Rehabilitation of the repaired ACL is a long process. A dancer requires fine control and extreme ranges as part of their normal activity. The use of tapes and braces when returning to dance is outside most aspects of performance.

Rehabilitation for a dancer post-ACL reconstruction will be broken down into four key stages (although timelines on the various aspects of each phase may overlap):

- **Phase 1: Protect/optimal loading.** This phase can range from 2 to 4 weeks, depending on the type of surgery undertaken. It includes restoration of the range of movement post-surgery, maintaining of muscle mass where possible, and working on developing improvements in areas above and below the knee, including core stability. CPMs (continuous passive mobilization machines) are useful in this phase. Additionally, a heel prop with the knee supported can allow the knee to move gently into extension under the pull of gravity. Maintenance of muscle mass can be achieved through the use of isometric muscle contractions, potentially enhanced using blood flow restriction training. Additional muscle mass support can be achieved via electromyographic (EMG) stimulation. Manual therapy can include patella mobilization. Exit criteria for this phase include full extension at the knee and 130 degrees of knee flexion.

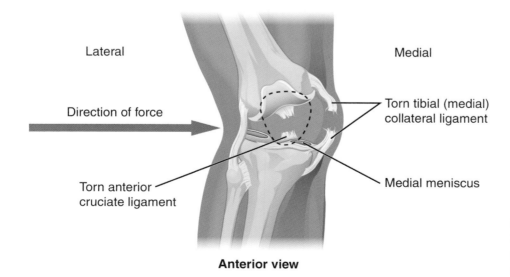

Anterior view

Fig. 34 Potential mechanism of injury for damage to ACL and MCL.

- **Phase 2: Core/proprioception/strength.** This phase builds on the work in Phase 1 and can run from week 4 until week 12. It sees the introduction of closed-chain exercises such as weight shifts and small squats. Loading can often be dependent on concomitant damage to either chondral surfaces or the meniscus and needs to be adjusted accordingly. This will also determine the time period for the use of crutches for walking. By week 6, in the absence of complications or concomitant pathology, there would be an expectation to be fully weight-bearing. There is also an increased emphasis on developing foundation proprioception in this phase. Strength work is still primarily dominated by closed-chain exercise delivery. A key feature of this phase is the increase of activity in the knee. A few key healing thresholds for ACL reconstructions are considered. Initial wound healing is important as it is a vulnerable period for infection. Typically, healing takes place within 2 weeks. Following suture removal, rehabilitation in water can take place. The next key period is the 6-week mark. At this point, healing is taking place within the bone tissue around the graft and screws, and an increase in activity is generally seen. As such, there may also be an increase in discomfort in the patient – warning the patient in advance may help to alleviate fears associated with this. It is typical, but it does need to be monitored carefully. Any increased intracapsular swelling might be an indication of the failure of the joint to tolerate the load experienced. In this case, the rehabilitation programme and the suitability of the advocated loading should be re-evaluated.
- **Phase 3: Dynamic proprioception/plyometric development/functional strength and power.** This phase sees the introduction of dynamic proprioception drills, which can be combined with plyometric exercises with 'hop and hold' drills. The use of unanticipated proprioception drills is also important. This can range from catch and throw drills while on a balance board, to shift the patient's centre of gravity, to destabilizing a BOSU ball while the patient stands flat side up.

Plyometric development can be broken down into key phases, from potential energy development in a jump preparation phase, to ballistic take-off and landing drills. This phase also introduces aspects of technical development, with dance-specific drills and programmes. Functional strength and power are supported through the development of strength and power endurance, with extended work phases and reduced rest phases. A strength or power endurance phase may mimic a typical dance solo piece, which might involve around two and a half minutes of high-intensity dancing. Using such time guidelines to develop high-intensity drills will better prepare the dancer for their functional requirements.

- **Phase 4: Functional integration.** This phase would be any time between 4 and 6 months. The longer-term impact of major injuries is better appreciated now, and there is a greater understanding of the risk of secondary changes affecting quality of life post-retirement. Clearly, any return to dance programme must allow sufficient time for the dancer to rehabilitate fully. As a result, the traditional time period may need to be extended from 6 months to 9 months. At this point the use of exit criteria, such as limb symmetry index testing, allows the development of 'dance fitness' through engagement in class, rehearsals and, ultimately, performances. Load, intensity and technical requirements can vary considerably with different repertoire and shows, and any decision relating to return to dance needs to consider these variables. Maintenance programmes for strength and power need to be continued through this period. Often it is useful to inform patients that the knee will take around 18 months to start feeling 'normal' again, and ensure that they understand the need to support and maintain it, with complementary programmes such as strength and power.

Return to dance following ACL reconstruction needs to examine the required level of function and consider the risk of recurrence, performance risk or

CASE STUDY 4: RETURN TO DANCE FOLLOWING ANTERIOR CRUCIATE LIGAMENT RECONSTRUCTION

The specific exercises referenced are given in Tables 23–28.

Table 22   Anterior cruciate ligament reconstruction rehabilitation plan.

WEEK	1	2	3	4	5	6	7–12	12–16	16–20	20+
Unload/core and range of movement										
Activate ankle plantar flexion/dorsiflexion (2x daily)	•	•								
Isometric quads/EMG stimulus (2x day)	•	•								
Knee slides (flex/ext/CPM) (every hour)	•	•								
Heel prop (passive knee extension), sitting (passive knee flex) (10 min every hour)	•	•	•							
Core session 1 (daily)	•	•	•							
Core/proprioception/strength										
Core session 2 (daily)			•	•	•	•				
Proprioception session 1 (daily)			•	•	•	•				
Introduction to strength session 1 (daily)				•	•	•	Alt day to Strength 1	Alt day to Strength 1	Alt day to Strength 1	Alt day to Strength 1
Hydrotherapy			•	•	•	Pool barre	Jump prep			
Strength session 1 (3x week am/pm)							•	•	•	•
Power/ground reaction force/dynamic proprioception										
Introduction to power session 1 (daily)							•	•	•	•
Power session 1 (3 x week)								•	•	•
Technical coaching (daily)								•	•	•
Functional integration										
Class									•	•
Rehearsal										•
Performance										•

Table 23   Core exercises.

	Reps	Sets	Rest
Core session 1			
Abductor isometric squeeze (0/45/90deg)	3×6–10sec hold/range	3	6–10sec
Sharman obliques	8–12	3	30sec
Sharman heel taps (within range of hip)	8–12	3	30sec
Isometric short clams @30-deg hip flex(with resistance band)	8–12	3	30sec
Isometric long clams @10-deg hip ext (with ankle weight if req.)	8–12	3	30sec
Prone hip extension (iso hold end range for 5 secs)	8–12	3	30sec
Bent-knee fall-outs	8–12	3	30sec

Table 24   Further core exercises.

	Reps	Sets	Rest
Core session 2			
Swiss ball prone/supine lateral roll-outs	8–12/position	2	30sec
Swiss ball 'plank' with single-leg lifts	8–12	2	30sec
Swiss ball bridge (shoulders on ball, hips/knees @ 90deg)	8–12	2	30sec
Swiss ball hamstring bridge (feet on ball, knees @ 30deg)	8–12	3	30sec
Swiss ball jack knife	8–12	3	30sec
Swiss ball hamstring pulls	9–12	3	30sec
Swiss ball sprinter's drill	8–12	3	30sec

Table 25   Strength exercises preparation.

	Reps	Sets	Rest
Preparation for strength session			
Heel rise	15–25	4	30sec
Body weight squat holds (15 sec holds)	12–15	3	30sec
Reverse glut/hamstring raise	12–15	3	30sec
Single-leg squat to rise	12–15	3	30sec
Single-leg 3-way reach/standing superman with med ball	12–15	3	30sec
Single-leg squat on unstable surface	12–15	3	30sec
Lunge on to unstable surface	12–15	3	30sec
Resisted turn (single-leg)	12–15	3	30sec
Body weight lateral squats (progress to load)	12–15	3	30sec
In-line cable wood chop	12–15	3	30sec
Dynamic wood chop with weighted plate	12–15	3	30sec
Crab walk out with resistance band	25 metres	4	30sec
Waiter's bow/good mornings	12–15	3	30sec

(continued overleaf)

CASE STUDY 4: RETURN TO DANCE FOLLOWING ANTERIOR CRUCIATE LIGAMENT RECONSTRUCTION *(continued)*

Table 26   Strength exercises.

	Reps	Sets	Rest
Strength session 1 (a.m.)			
Romanian dead lift	3–6	5	1min
Loaded side-lying hip internal rotation (hip 90deg)	3–6	5	1min
Loaded side-lying hip external rotation (hip 90deg)	3–6	5	1min
Sumo squats	3–6	5	1min
Bulgarian split squats	3–6	5	1min
Hammer press with forward step	8–12	3	1min
Strength session 1 (p.m.)	**Reps**	**Sets**	**Rest**
Front squats	3–6	5	1min
Loaded hip extension/thrusts	3–6	5	1min
Sumo squats	3–6	5	1min
Lateral squat	3–6	5	1min
Turkish get up	8–12	3	1min

Table 27   Power exercises introduction.

	Reps	Sets	Rest
Introduction to power session 1			
Heel rise with ballistic rebound	8–12	3	30sec
Reformer jump drills	8–12	3	30sec
Ladder drills – travelling with hops and cross-overs	15 metres	4	30sec
Hop and holds	8–12	3	30sec
Mini hurdle drills (forwards, sideways)	15 metres	4	30sec

Table 28   Power exercises.

	Reps	Sets	Rest
Power session 1			
Pogos	30 sec	1	30sec
Hop and hold (front and back)	6–8	1	30sec
Hop and hold (lateral)	6–8	1	30sec
Squat jumps	6–8	1	30sec
Lateral squat rebound jumps	6–8	1	30sec
Split squat jumps	6–8	1	30sec
Jump box explosive jumps (2 leg to 2 legs)	6–8	1	1 min
Jump box explosive jumps (2 leg to 1 leg)	6–8	1	1 min
Jump box explosive jumps (1 leg to 2 legs)	6–8	1	1 min
Jump box explosive jumps (1 leg to 1 legs)	6–8	1	1 min
Jump box controlled landing (2 legs to 2 legs)	6–8	1	1 min
Jump box controlled landing (2 legs to 1 leg)	6–8	1	1 min
Hang cleans	6–8	4	1–2 min

secondary changes in later life if insufficiently reha-bilitated. The literature suggests many reasons as to why ACL patients fail to return to previous levels of participation in pivoting and contact sports. Some are non-modifiable, such as age and gender, some are associated with the surgical process and deci-sion making, including graft type and placement, and some are associated with the rehabilitation process, including decisions on return to the vary-ing levels of activity and full return criteria.

It is advocated that time (or biological) as well as functional criteria be used when determining a suit-able time to return to dance, to ensure a reduced risk of re-injury. Functional criteria can include a multi-tude of parameters, both physical (clinical and phys-iological-based assessments) and psychological.

Physiological-based testing may include strength (isometric, isokinetic), neuromuscular and prop-rioceptive, dynamic tests. They may be based on pre-established values from screening protocols or using the limb symmetry index approach. Functional tests could include a technical session assessing alignment and control through key movements, progressing on to pivoting and jumping drills.

Significant demands are often placed on a dancer for their return to dance. However, research has demonstrated that delaying a return to full activity in sports by 3 more months, from 6 months to 9 months, led to a reduced risk of re-injury of 51 per cent for each month the return was delayed. Given the role of the ACL in pivot stability and the nature of pivoting in dance, this needs careful considera-tion. Presently, evidence from sport suggests that a strength deficit of greater than 25 per cent will increase the risk of re-injury, and a strength deficit of greater than 10 per cent may result in a perform-ance deficit as tested through isokinetic testing of quadricep and hamstrings. If a dancer has access to functional testing, isokinetic strength testing can be a useful adjunct in return-to-dance deci-sion-making. Power testing is also important. This might be force plate or jump mat testing, or simple distance and time hop tests, comparing affected and unaffected limbs. Given the increased risk of secondary changes in later life, it is the responsibil-ity of the health professional to give returning danc-ers clear information about how a return that is too early might have an impact on that risk.

Joint Injuries of the Knee

Often associated with ACL injuries, but also encoun-tered in isolation, injuries to the articular cartilage and meniscus can be either traumatic or long-term. A traumatic injury might occur with the sheering of the femoral condyle over the tibial plateau follow-ing an awkward land, for example. A longer-term injury might happen through repeated loading over time, coupled with less than optimal biomechan-ics. Damage to a dancer's articular cartilage can be seen in the femoral condyles, typically the medial compartment, as well as the retro-patella surface; again, the medial facet region is typically damaged. It is critical in the management of articular cartilage damage to correct any biomechanical patterns that may have created the overload. Given the vulner-ability of the medial compartment, control of the femoral anteversion, through adequate control of the proximal external rotators of the hip as well as navicular drop/pronation of the foot, is key. These may be tackled through isolation drills composing of isometric or eccentric control, or through func-tional training focusing on movement competency and landing mechanics.

Medical management of articular damage in the knee may involve the use of repeated hyaluronic acid injections, to reduce pain and support joint surfaces. This is an alternative to corticosteroids, which may over time have a negative impact on joint surface integrity. Surgical management can involve the stabilization of the outer edges of a defect, the stimulation of new cell growth with micro-fracturing techniques, or cell transplantation with mosaic-plasty procedures. Rehabilitation following surgical intervention is a lengthy process, particularly where micro-fracturing or transplantation procedures have been undertaken, requiring cell growth and stabili-zation. Typically, these patients will progress to full weight-bearing within 3 months, but must always be aware of supporting the immature cartilage cells. Maintenance of range of movement and muscle

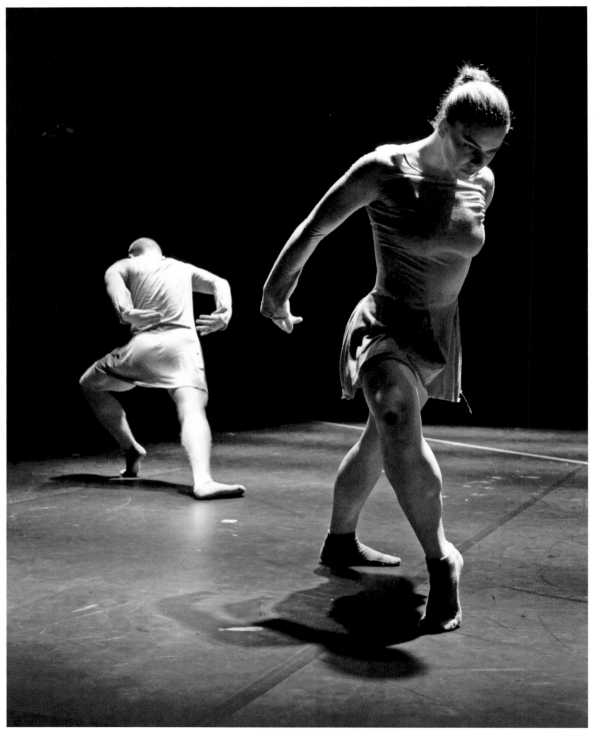

Photo 101   Many dance choreographies may place the knee at risk, including jumps and rotational knee bend positions.

mass in the early stages is challenging and the use of continuous passive mobilization (CPMs) is an important adjunct. The use of electro-muscular stimulation may also benefit. Once the cartilage is consolidated, rehabilitation can focus on strength restoration, followed by strength endurance. Power and power endurance work follow predetermined exit criteria, typically achieving a limb symmetry of within 25 per cent in strength testing. Functional integration and return to dance in surgical candidates may be from 9 to 12 months post-surgery. As with ACL return-to-dance timelines, there is a good correlation between the longer rehabilitation time and long-term outcomes, with dancers able to return to full function and continue a professional career for many years following surgery. The temptation to rush dancers back following surgery needs to be avoided, as it may have a significant impact on both the length of their career and the quality of life in later years.

Like chondral defects, meniscal damage can occur as a result of overuse or trauma. Again, as in chondral damage, correction of any abnormal biomechanics is critical to a successful long-term return to dance. When assessing a ballet dancer with a suspected meniscal tear, it is important to evaluate their turn-out technique, to ensure that they are not rotating the lower leg in an effort to enhance the effect. This causes excessive torsion through the knee, which may over time lead to degenerative changes and a vulnerability of the meniscal cartilage and, ultimately, the articular cartilage. The position of the tear may influence management decisions. If the tear extends into the red zone (the outer edge of the meniscus), there is a better chance of healing, as there is a good blood supply. In this case, every effort should be made to preserve the meniscus, whether via a medical or surgical route. When managing a dancer with a meniscal tear, it is preferable to avoid steroid injection to manage pain and the associated intracapsular swelling, as part of a longer-term strategy of the preserving articular cartilage. Platelet-rich plasma (PRP) has been used successfully in the medical management of chronic meniscal tears, alongside a rehabilitation programme to correct femoral loading and overall strength and stability. Surgical management of meniscal tears via arthroscopy has offered patients quick turn-around potentials, particularly in meniscectomy as opposed to repair procedures. With the increase in point pressure on the articular cartilage following the removal of a section of meniscus, it is imperative to do more to improve biomechanics and unloading of the knee joint in response to forces. This may be achieved through adequate strength and power development.

Although it has a low prevalence in dance, the risk to the patella from direct trauma needs to be considered. Contemporary choreography may entail landing directly on the knee, risking potential patella fracture. Management of patella fractures can be conservative if the extensor mechanism is intact, but warrants an orthopaedic opinion. The risk of patella subluxation or dislocation also exists within dance. Although patella dislocations may spontaneously relocate, the risk of damage to the medial patella femoral ligament (MPFL) needs close assessment to establish its overall stability and chance of recurrence. Many first-time dislocations can be managed conservatively if there is an absence of an osteochondral fracture or disruption of the MPFL. An orthopaedic opinion should be sought in the case of recurrent dislocations. Rehabilitation of post-surgical patella dislocation follows a similar programme to that advocated after ACL surgery, but with more emphasis on the medial knee stabilizers instead of the hamstrings (which are emphasized in the ACL programme).

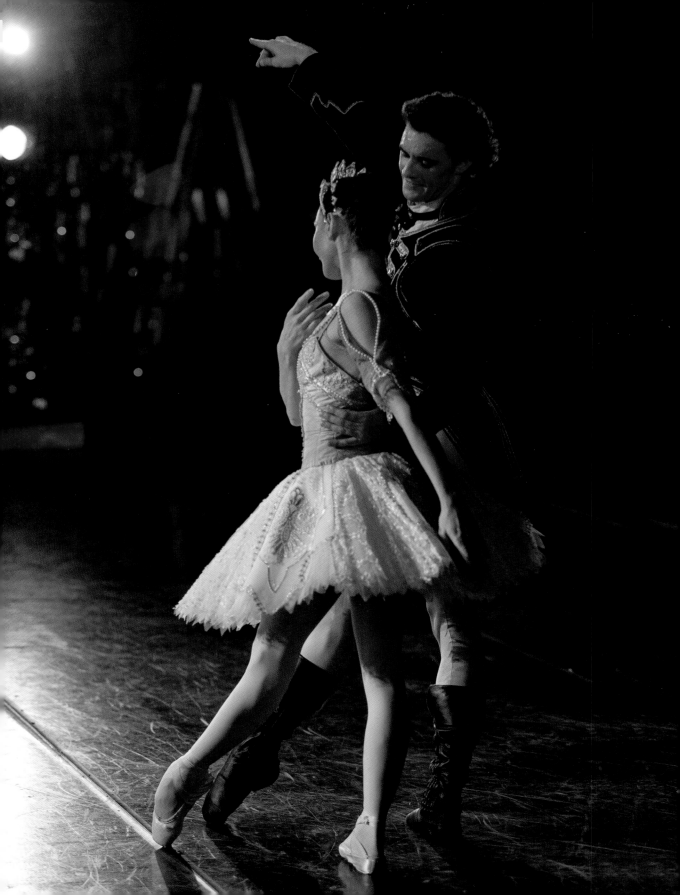

CHAPTER 10

LOWER LEG, ANKLE AND FOOT INJURIES

Many of the published epidemiological studies relating to dance report that the highest incidence of injuries occurs in the lower leg, ankle and foot. Given the nature of dance, a good understanding of the anatomy and biomechanics of this region is vital in addressing the injuries sustained by dancers. Loading through the tibia in dance sees the potential for an adaptive change in the anterior cortex, which is a means to support the tibia against the loading patterns in dance but inadvertently creates a vulnerability to injury, namely anterior tibial cortex stress fractures. This is a challenging pathology to manage in any athletic population. Dancers are also susceptible to the more common ankle and foot injuries, including lateral ligament sprains, avulsion fractures and tendon issues. The high exposure rates seen in dance give rise to subtle loading patterns of the ankle and foot. Over time, this may cause a slight change to the optimal biomechanics, which can eventually manifest in injury. Success in the management of these cases will come from an intricate understanding of biomechanics and the ability to influence loading patterns through small changes.

LOWER LEG

Anatomy and Associated Pathology

Like the upper leg, the lower leg consists of three compartments (anterolateral, lateral and posterior),

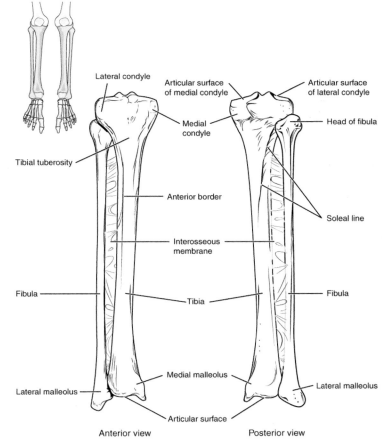

Lateral condyle
Articular surface of medial condyle
Medial condyle
Tibial tuberosity
Anterior border
Interosseous membrane
Fibula
Tibia
Medial malleolus
Lateral malleolus
Articular surface

Articular surface of lateral condyle
Head of fibula
Soleal line
Fibula
Lateral malleolus

Anterior view   Posterior view

Fig. 35 Bony anatomy of the lower leg.

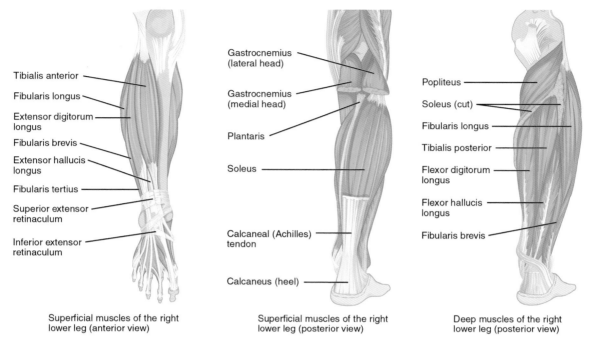

Tibialis anterior

Fibularis longus

Extensor digitorum longus

Fibularis brevis

Extensor hallucis longus

Fibularis tertius

Superior extensor retinaculum

Inferior extensor retinaculum

Gastrocnemius (lateral head)

Gastrocnemius (medial head)

Plantaris

Soleus

Calcaneal (Achilles) tendon

Calcaneus (heel)

Popliteus

Soleus (cut)

Fibularis longus

Tibialis posterior

Flexor digitorum longus

Flexor hallucis longus

Fibularis brevis

Superficial muscles of the right lower leg (anterior view)

Superficial muscles of the right lower leg (posterior view)

Deep muscles of the right lower leg (posterior view)

Fig. 36   Muscular anatomy of the lower leg.

separated by the interosseous membrane and the two long bones of the lower leg, the tibia and fibula. The compartments contain the muscles outside the foot that provide movement through the foot and ankle.

The anterolateral compartment contains the tibialis anterior, extensor hallucis and extensor digitorum, all of which serve as dorsiflexors. With the predominance of plantar flexion in dance movements, there is typically a low prevalence of injuries to muscles in the anterolateral compartment.

The lateral compartment houses the peroneal longus and brevis muscles. Although, due to their origin and insertion, they can act as weak plantar flexors, it is their role as evertors and ankle stabilizers that is important in dance. Ankle sprains are the most prevalent injury in dance and there is a reported prevalence of chronic instability following ankle sprains generally, so the role of these muscles and their response to injury is important.

The posterior compartment is further divided into a deep and superficial component. The tibialis

posterior, flexor hallucis longus and flexor digitorum longus muscles sit in the deep portion of the posterior compartment. This is one of the most important considerations for an attending clinician, particularly when examining ballet dancers. The tendons of these muscles track behind the medial malleoli and can invert the foot and flex the toes. The tibialis posterior is also known as a plantar flexor of the foot, notably in the initiation of the heel lift. Gastrocnemius, soleus and plantaris are found in the superficial component of the posterior compartment.

The tendinous insertion of the triceps surae (made up of gastrocnemius and soleus), the Achilles tendon, is vulnerable to overuse injuries in the form of tendinosis and tendinopathy. As such, this region is an important consideration in dance. Posterior lower leg pain is also associated with popliteal artery insufficiency, where the patient reports increased calf pain on exertion. Popliteal artery insufficiency can be as a result of an atypical arterial pathway, atypical muscle origin, or a combination of both. Although it is considered to have a very low preva-

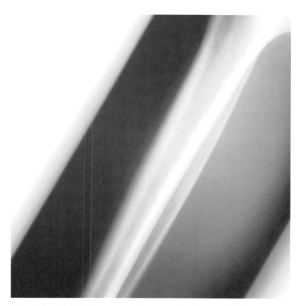

Fig. 37 Plain film x-ray demonstrating a thickened anterior cortex of the tibia. There are also faint linear translucencies, suggesting anterior tibial cortex stress fractures.

lence, it should be considered with exertional calf pain, given the prevalence of hypertrophy in the calf musculature of some dancers.

The tibia is the key weight-bearing bone while the fibula's role is primarily for muscle attachment. The nature of loading through a dancer's lower leg, particularly in ballet and with repeated plié or small knee bend movements, leads to a risk of an adaptive thickening of the anterior cortex of the tibia.

Any thickening of the cortex, while part of the protective adaptation to loading, may also lead to an increased risk of developing an anterior cortex stress response or fracture. Although its prevalence may be lower than that of, for example, an ankle sprain, a bone-stress injury can be severe, requiring a significant amount of time to resolve, thus delaying a return to dance. As such, it needs to be considered a high-risk injury. These injuries typically can occur in the proximal third of the tibia, and may take the form of a single defined fracture or multiple fractures. Management of an anterior tibial cortex stress fracture is a challenging process, over a prolonged

period. Correction of biomechanics is paramount. Posterior chain muscle conditioning allows a shift of the centre of pressure and can reduce the loading impact on the anterior tibial cortex. In combination with an improvement of the ankle mechanics, through anterior and usually posterior tibial muscle support, symptoms can be reduced and a full return to dance activities facilitated.

Medial Tibial Stress Syndrome

The medial border of the tibia is another vulnerable region for dancers. The incidence of medial tibial stress syndrome (MTSS) can be high in many genres, including ballet. Medial lower leg pain can be categorized as follows:

- **Type 1: Tibial microfracture, bone stress reaction or cortical fracture.** A similar management approach to the anterior tibial stress fracture can be adopted, with focus on offloading the lower leg to a degree where symptoms are not experienced in the healing phase. The secondary phase involves correcting causative factors such as strength, biomechanics and technique, and the final phase can concentrate on consolidating power and power endurance alongside technical endurance.
- **Type 2: Periostealgia.** As with a stress fracture, it is key to examine biomechanics and address any technical areas that may predispose the region to excessive loading. Eccentric internal rotation control of the hip/femur alongside eccentric control of the tibialis posterior in controlling navicular drop is paramount.
- **Type 3: Chronic compartment syndrome.** The overdevelopment of musculature in the lower leg can result in ischemic vascular compromise during exercise. Symptoms are almost exclusively bilateral. The level of pain is disproportionately high during exercise but it will typically fully resolve with no residual symptoms within 30 minutes of finishing. Diagnosis is made through compartment pressure testing. This is an invasive procedure, so a clear working diagnosis is needed before commencing. Management is

Table 29 Rehabilitation of medial tibial stress syndrome.

Exercise and progression	Description: session A (perform 2× day, 3× week)	Progressive overload		
		Reps per set	Sets	Rest between sets
1. Side-lying isometric hip extension		3–5/leg with 7 sec hold	2	3sec between contract
2. Side-lying isometric hip ext rotation		3–5/leg with 7 sec hold	2	3sec between contract
3. Swiss ball straight-leg bridge (SL)	Feet on Swiss ball, lying flat on back	10–12	2	30sec
4. Swiss ball reverse bridge (SL)	Shoulders on Swiss ball	10–12	2	30sec
5. Side-lying leg lift (int rot)	5 sec hold – possibly add small ankle weight (2kg)	6–8	3	30sec
6. Side-lying leg lift (ext rot)	5 sec hold – possibly add small ankle weight (2kg)	6–8	3	30sec
7. 'Over a step' tib post drops	Emphasis on flattening and arching the medial longitudinal arch	6–8	3	30sec
8. Heel rise with tib post bias	Heel rise with theraband pulling at 45deg medially	15–25	2	30sec
9. Foot rises (beats)	Heels placed 30cm from wall leaning back into wall, pressure and weight-bearing on heels – pull foot/toes upwards (dorsiflexion), control back to ground	10–12	2–3	30sec
10. Heel 'hop and holds'	Like a typical hop and hold but instructed to 'land' hop on the heels and control the foot so as not to touch the floor	10	2/leg	30sec

surgical fasciotomy. A more recent classification system has used MRI, with the emphasis on bony reaction. The Fredericson MTSS Classification System from MRI delineates the degree of periosteal and cortical bone involvement in a scale from 0 (normal) to 4b (a region of intercortical signal change). These classifications have been purported to assist in timeline prediction for return to activity.

Rehabilitation of MTSS must strike a balance between load and biomechanical adjustments. The ability to unload sufficiently to facilitate appropriate muscle firing patterns. Correction of biomechanics needs to account for the proximal control achieved from the hip, as well local control to withstand the eccentric loading of the tibialis posterior as the foot controls against overpronation and navicular drop.

An example of a programme for MTSS is shown in Table 29.

ANKLE AND FOOT

Anatomy and Associated Pathology

Given the role of the ankle and the foot in dance, it is no surprise that ankle injuries are reported to be the most prevalent in dancers. One key feature of most sports is the ability of the body to travel over a planted foot, as in running. Dance is no different. For the torso to pass over the foot, it is dependent on three key pivot points through the foot and ankle: the round underside of the calcaneus, dorsiflexion through the ankle joint and dorsiflexion through the metatarsal phalangeal joints. In addition to this, the various joints through the foot and ankle contribute to the overall function.

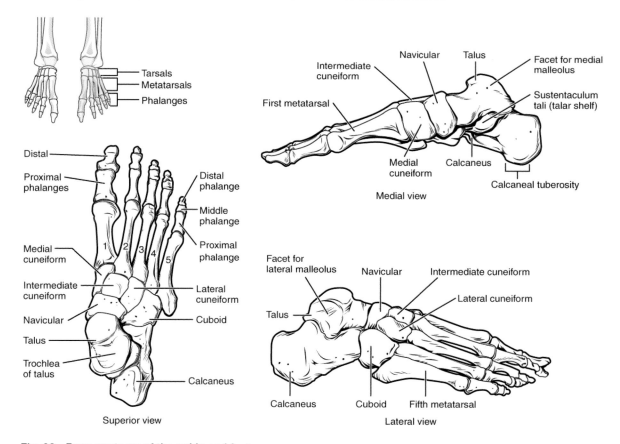

Fig. 38   Bony anatomy of the ankle and foot.

The talocrural joint is a primary torque convertor as well as allowing for a small degree of transverse and frontal movement. The bony morphology provides a notable degree of the stability of the joint, particularly in the talocrural neutral position. Patients who are subject to a forceful inversion in this position may sustain a fracture dislocation, due to the shape and position of the talus and lateral malleoli. The subtalar joint provides the secondary torque converter, with postural adjustments into pronation and supination taking place through this joint. When the torso travels over the planted foot, the dorsiflexion needed is achieved through the axis of the malleoli. There is an obliquity of this axis that produces relative lateral deviation in dorsiflexion. To facilitate this movement there is a need for the fibula to move laterally and cephalically. The absence of this can produce a risk of anterolateral synovitis. When the ankle passes into plantar flexion, there is a degree of relative medial deviation, due to the obliquity of the ankle's axis.

These movements and the role of the subtalar joint combine through the gait cycle where, during midstance to toe-off phase, the heel is everted at the subtalar joint and the forefoot is pronated to be loaded, as the weight-bearing is transferred to the first and second metatarsal phalangeal joints. As this region is the final pivot point, restrictions seen in conditions such as hallux limitus become an important part of an assessment process.

The foot and ankle region are heavily supported by ligaments, muscles and tendons as part of its stabilization and locomotor function. Due to the higher prevalence of inversion injuries, there is an increased need to understand its structural and functional supports. The lateral ankle is supported by three key ligaments that make up the lateral ligament complex. The anterior talofibular ligament (ATFL) becomes taut when the ankle is in plantar flexion and acts as a collateral ligament. In an ankle neutral position, the ATFL resists anterior displacement of the talus and rotational displacement of the tibia. The calcaneofibular ligament (CFL) tightens in dorsiflexion and acts as a collateral ligament as well as providing stability of the subtalar joint. The posterior talofibular (PTFL) provides support against inversion in the presence of a deficient CFL and rotation in the presence of a deficient ATFL. The lateral complex is further supported by the presence of the talonavicular and calcaneocuboid ligaments.

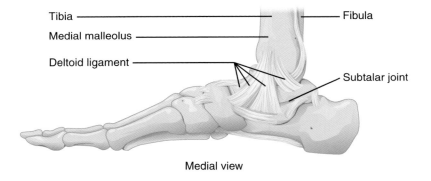

Tibia ——————————— Fibula
Medial malleolus ——————
Deltoid ligament ——————
Subtalar joint

Medial view

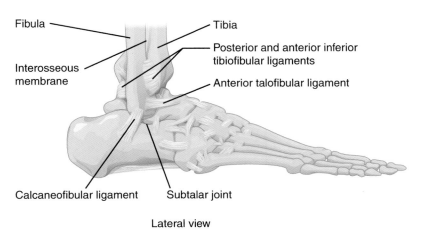

Fibula ——
Interosseous membrane ——
Tibia
Posterior and anterior inferior tibiofibular ligaments
Anterior talofibular ligament
Calcaneofibular ligament — Subtalar joint

Lateral view

Fig. 39 Ligamentous anatomy of the ankle and foot.

Although they are not always considered part of the static stabilizers, the presence of the peroneal tendons provides both static and dynamic stability for the lateral ankle. As dynamic stabilizers, the peroneals provide resistance against inversion in a plantar flexed position of the ankle. The insertion of peroneal brevis into the base of the fifth supports its action as both abductor and pronator of the anterior aspect of the forefoot. Peroneal longus runs alongside peroneus brevis up to the cuboid bone, where it passes obliquely to the medial cuneiform and first metatarsal. The insertion facilitates its critical role of stabilization of the plantar arches. This is further supported through the plantar insertions of tibialis posterior. While other athletic populations may make use of orthotic inserts to support the arches of the foot, these are generally not suitable in dance, with dancers performing in ballet flats or pointe shoes, jazz shoes, or even barefoot. As the ability to employ additional support is restricted in this way, it is vital to utilize all aspects of muscular support for the arch of the foot.

Given the role of ligaments as mechanoreceptors, a laxity in them can result in a latency in the contraction of the peroneals. This can lead to an occurrence of an inversion ankle sprain. The medial ankle has similar layers of support. The medial ligament complex or deltoid ligament complex is made of the posterior tibiotalar ligament, tibiocalcaneal ligament and the tibionavicular ligament. There are both deep and superficial layers. As the deep fibres cannot be palpated, assessment of the area is based on looking at the stability of the talus, further supported by results of any imaging.

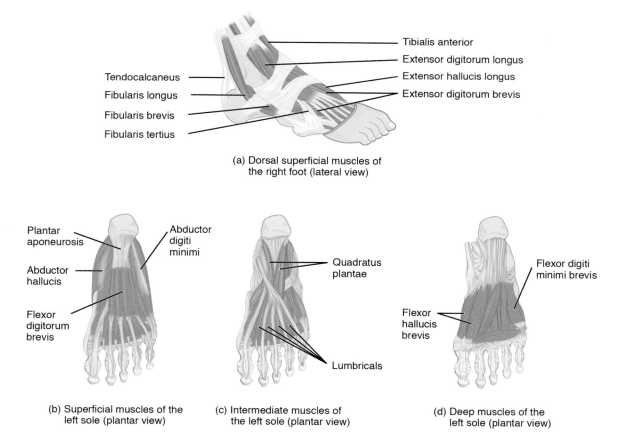

Tibialis anterior
Extensor digitorum longus
Extensor hallucis longus
Extensor digitorum brevis
Tendocalcaneus
Fibularis longus
Fibularis brevis
Fibularis tertius

(a) Dorsal superficial muscles of the right foot (lateral view)

Plantar aponeurosis
Abductor digiti minimi
Abductor hallucis
Flexor digitorum brevis

(b) Superficial muscles of the left sole (plantar view)

Quadratus plantae
Lumbricals

(c) Intermediate muscles of the left sole (plantar view)

Flexor digiti minimi brevis
Flexor hallucis brevis

(d) Deep muscles of the left sole (plantar view)

Figs 40a–d Muscular anatomy of the ankle and foot.

CASE STUDY 5: ACUTE ANKLE SPRAIN IN DANCE

A professional female ballet dancer underwent a Brostrom reconstruction of her ATFL following a traumatic rupture from an awkward landing of a jump. A balance is needed between biological timelines associated with good healing of the graft (typically a restriction of up to 6 weeks into plantar flexion) and the required range of movement. Furthermore, it is important to consolidate strength as the range develops. For these reasons, a rehabilitation programme may be extended to 6 months. The period is broken into biological timelines as follows:

1. 2 weeks of protection with the ankle unloaded and elevated;

Table 30   Acute ankle sprain rehabilitation plan.

WEEK	1–2	3–4	5–6	7–11	12–18	19–26
Unload/core and range of movement						
Elevation, non-weight-bearing	•					
Elevation, partial weight-bearing	•	•	•			
Sitting knee extensions – isometric, straight-leg raise and small knee bends (every 2 hours)	•	•	•			
Ankle active and passive dorsiflexion (plantar flexion from week 6) (every 2 hours)		•	•(pf)	•		
Ankle isometric contractions – all directions (every 2 hours)		•	•			
Core session 1 (2× day)		•	•			
Core/proprioception/strength						
Proprioception session 1				•	•	
Gait walking drills (high knees and backwards)				•		
Introduction to strength session 1 (daily)				•	•	
Core session 2				•	•	•
Proprioception session 2					•	•
Strength session 1 (2× day, 3× week)					•	•
Jump proprioception/ground reaction force/functional strength						
Foot rise (progress to beats)					•	•
Introduction to power session 1 (daily, alternate days when starting power session 1)					•	•
Pool barre					•	
Pool jumps					•	
Power session (3 × week)					•	•
Technical coaching					•	•
Functional integration						
Class (barre and centre initially)					•	•
Rehearsal						•
Performance						•

2. 4 weeks spent focusing on regaining range of movement where allowed (as indicated, plantar flexion may be restricted in the first 6 weeks);

3. around 6 weeks of obtaining full range of movement as well as starting initial proprioception and strength work;

4. a 6-week block consolidating strength and proprioception as well as introducing power work and technical work, including preparation for pointe work;

5. the final 6- to 8-week period involves consolidation of power and develops strength and power endurance, as well as allowing time to regain full functional fitness through participation in dance activities such as class and rehearsals.

A further challenge occasionally encountered with female dancers is the concern over hypertrophying through the rehabilitation process. With this in mind, the strength sessions do not use typical reps and sets based around the 80–100 per cent 1RM. Where possible, the use of blood flow restriction training can create the desired physiological impact. If it is not tolerated or is contraindicated, the use of 'time under load' can develop the functional strength required. This may, however, mean an extension to the overall timelines, in order to allow sufficient time for the physiological adaptation to training.

The specific exercises referenced are given in Tables 31–38.

Table 31 Core exercises.

	Reps	Sets	Rest
Core session 1			
Abductor isometric squeeze (0/45/90deg)	3×6–10sec hold/range	3	6–10sec
Sahrmann's obliques	8×6–10sec hold/range	3	10sec
Sahrmann's heel taps	8–12	3	30sec
Resisted clams	8–12	3	30sec
Side-lying clock	8–12	3	30sec
Prone hip extension	8–12	3	30sec
Bent knee fall-outs	8–12	3	30sec

Table 32 Core exercises.

	Reps	Sets	Rest
Core session 2			
Swiss ball roll-outs	8–12	3	30sec
Swiss ball bridge	8–12	3	30sec
Swiss ball hamstring bridge	8–12	3	30sec
Swiss ball jack knife	8–12	3	30sec
Swiss ball sprinter's drill	8–12	3	30sec

CASE STUDY 5: ACUTE ANKLE SPRAIN IN DANCE *(continued)*

Table 33   Proprioception exercises.

	Reps	Sets	Rest
Proprioception session 1			
Eyes open stretch mat	6×10sec hold	3	10sec
Eyes closed stretch mat (support as needed)	6×10sec hold	3	10sec
Eyes open AIRex mat	6×10sec hold	3	10sec
Eyes closed AIRex mat (support as needed)	6×10sec hold	3	10sec
BIODEX limits of stability (close target)	3×1min 3 targets	2	1min

Table 34   Further proprioception exercises.

	Reps	Sets	Rest
Proprioception session 2			
Single-leg squat to rise	8–12	3	30sec
Single-leg 3-way reach with rise	8–12	3	30sec
Single-leg squat on unstable surface	8–12	3	30sec
Lunge on to unstable surface	8–12	3	30sec
Unstable turn-out	8–12	3	30sec
Backwards lunge on to unstable surface	8–12	3	30sec

Table 35   Strength exercises introduction.

	Reps	Sets	Rest
Introduction to strength session 1			
Resistance band push and pull	15–25	4	30sec
Pool plié to rise – progress to turn-out	15–25	4	30sec
Reformer plié to rise – progress to turn-out	15–25	4	30sec

Table 36   Strength exercises.

	Reps	Sets	Rest
Strength session 1			
Body weight squats	8–12	3	30sec
Body weight lateral squats	8–12	3	30sec
In-line wood chop cable	8–12	3	30sec
Dynamic wood chop	8–12	3	30sec
Crab walk out with turn-out	10m × 2	4	30sec
Heel rise (with isometric inversion with resistance band)	15–25	4	30sec

Table 37   Power exercises introduction.

	Reps	Sets	Rest
Introduction to power session 1			
Heel rise with ballistic rebound	8–12	3	30sec
Reformer jump drills	8–12	3	30sec
Ladder drills – travelling with hops and cross-overs	15 metres	4	30sec
Hop and hold	8–12	3	30sec
Mini hurdle drills (forwards, sideways)	15 metres	4	30sec

Table 38   Power exercises.

	Reps	Sets	Rest
Power session 1			
Pogos	30 sec	1	30sec
Hop and hold (front and back)	6–8	1	30sec
Hop and hold (lateral)	6–8	1	30sec
Squat jumps	6–8	1	30sec
Lateral squat rebound jumps	6–8	1	30sec
Split squat jumps	6–8	1	30sec
Jump box explosive jumps (2 leg to 2 legs)	6–8	1	1 min
Jump box explosive jumps (2 leg to 1 leg)	6–8	1	1 min
Jump box explosive jumps (1 leg to 2 legs)	6–8	1	1 min
Jump box explosive jumps (1 leg to 1 legs)	6–8	1	1 min
Jump box controlled landing (2 legs to 2 legs)	6–8	1	1 min
Jump box controlled landing (2 legs to 1 leg)	6–8	1	1 min

Table 39   Ankle mobility programme.

Exercise and progression	Description: Ankle mobility perform daily and pre- exercise	Progressive overload		
		Reps per set	Sets	Rest between sets
1. Plié posterior pull	Mulligan mobilization with movement (posterior fibula glide with band)	8–10	2–3	30sec
2. Foot rises (beats)	Heels placed 30cm from wall, leaning back into wall, pressure and weight-bearing on heels – pull foot/toes upwards (dorsiflexion), control back to ground	15–25	2–3	20-30sec
3. Heel rises	Standing over edge of step, ensuring weight-bearing through the first and second metatarsal heads, rise on to demi-pointe. Progress to single-leg	15–25	2–3	20–30sec
4. Pogos	Possibly on aero floor	15	1–3	30sec

Like the lateral complex, muscle tendons provide important static and dynamic stability through the tendons of tibialis posterior, flexor digitorum longus and flexor hallucis longus. Tibialis posterior plays an important role in both the initiation of plantarflexion from neutral as well as stabilization of the midfoot during toe-off. Tibialis posterior via multiple insertion points into the tarsal bones acts as the primary dynamic stabilizer of the rearfoot and the medial longitudinal arch in plantar flexion. The location of the tibialis posterior tendon relative to the axes of the subtalar and ankle joints facilitates inversion and plantarflexion respectively, and is the most powerful supinator of the hindfoot as a result of the large inverter moment arm acting on the subtalar joint. As the foot moves into pronation to allow weight-bearing through the first and second metatarsal heads, to facilitate toe-off during gait, the role of flexor halluces longus is important for stability and force propulsion.

Similarly, the hindfoot is well supported; some authors, including Cromeen in 2011, suggest that as many as 26 ligaments support this region. Key ligaments in the region include the posterior inferior tibiofibular ligament, along with the interosseous membrane, providing up to 30 per cent of the high ankle stability. Furthermore, reports of increased signal change of the inter-malleoli ligament on MRI suggest traumatic inflammatory changes in dancers with a positive posterior impingement test. Whether this represents an impact injury or a stressing of the ligament as the ankle mortise splays is unclear at this stage. It does, however, point to the relevance of creating stability and control of movement into the extremes of plantar flexion for dance.

As in most sports, lateral ligaments, particularly the ATFL, are more frequently injured than medial or syndesmotic ligaments. Grading systems are useful to describe the extent of ligament sprains. As the psychological impact of an injury for both recreational or elite dancers or athletes can be significant, the language used to describe that injury can have a notable impact on how they understand and process the information. Elite athletes and dancers are often already familiar with Grade 1, 2 or 3 ligament sprains. However, an avulsion fracture on a radiology report may need to be explained to the patient, in relation to the (ankle) sprain. Pain radiating from the sinus tarsi can be associated with inversion injuries. The sinus tarsi is a cone-shaped tunnel between the talus and the calcaneal bone, containing ligaments, nerves and blood vessels. T2 weighted MRI scans in suspected cases may confirm increased signal uptake. Its involvement in pain provocation can be further confirmed using a diagnostic anaesthetic injection with a pain provocation test. If successful, a local steroid injection can be used to address symptoms. The stability of the ankle complex (both medial and lateral) needs to be addressed as part of the overall management process.

Surgical reconstruction of the lateral ligament complex can result in a limitation of range. Dancers are required to achieve a supranatural range of plantar flexion for demi-pointe and pointe work, as well as dorsiflexion in pliés and grand pliés, so range of movement post-surgery is critical.

Chronic stiffness is always a risk post-surgery. Furthermore, the 'feel' of the ankle may not be the same for an extended period (anything up to 18 months) after reconstruction. An ankle mobility programme can be useful in creating a dynamic capacity in the joint. With the typical restrictions seen in dorsiflexion, due to the loss of fibular translation and normal 'gapping' seen at the mortise joint in this position, working on both the joint mobility and muscle activators is important.

Although it has a low prevalence, the position and impact of the interosseous membrane in the syndesomosis need to be considered in persistent anterior lateral pain and impingement. Typically, they present with pain in the absence of swelling. They can be insidious in onset. MRI scans tend to be normal but, when explored arthroscopically, the membrane is seen to be collapsed and impinging in the talocrural joint through dorsiflexion. This may be as a result of years of repeated forced plantar and dorsiflexion. Management involves removal of the impinging tissue followed by a rehabilitation process similar to that undertaken after syndesmotic ankle sprains.

Chronic Ankle Instability

Chronic instability of the ankle may be present in a dancer in the absence of notable trauma, having been acquired over the course of a career. The role of functional instability over mechanical instability is a key assessment. Associated with ankle pain following inversion injuries, pain may originate from the anterior lateral aspect of the ankle and the sinus tarsi. Sinus tarsi pain may also present in atraumatic functionally unstable ankles. While guided steroid injections may assist in reducing pain, a full stability programme is required for improved long-term results. Similarly, medial pain associated with loading of the plantar calcaneonavicular ligament (spring ligament) has been reported. With its attachment on the sustentaculum of the calcaneus and proximity to the groove on which the flexor hallucis runs over the sustentaculum tali, it is important to differentiate between tendon and ligament as well as the biomechanical stresses through the areas as a potential causative factor.

Ankle Posterior Impingement

There is also a strong correlation between increased range of movement through the ankle associated with lateral ankle instability and posterior impingement signs. While there is a reported higher prevalence of os trigonums in dancers, this is more likely to be associated with the ranges used for demi-pointe and pointe work, which utilize extremes of plantar flexion, creating the approximation of posterior ankle surfaces.

It is important with posterior impingement symptoms in dancers to establish whether they relate to a soft-tissue or bony impingement. Here, the clinical relevance of an os trigonum (accessory bone in the posterior recess) or steida process (elongated lateral tubercle of the posterior talus) is pertinent. An MRI is a useful adjunct to establish this. In the absence of bony involvement through an os trigonum or steida process, rest, relative offload of full plantar flexion with biomechanical adjustments (and possibly technical adjustments if the dancer

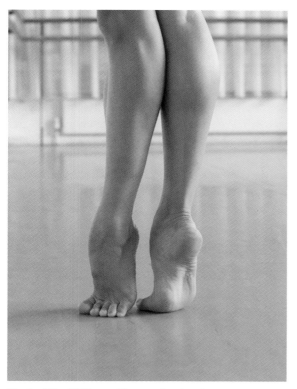

Photo 102   Fifth position en demi-pointe.

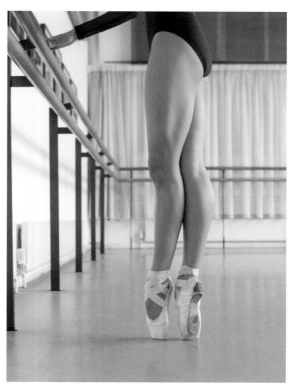

Photo 103   Fifth position en pointe.

over-plantarflexes their foot), and nonsteroidal anti-inflammatories (or, if it fails to respond, ultrasound guided steroid injection) can be very successful. The importance of correct accessory movement of the subtalar joint must not be underestimated in these cases. If an os trigonum is identified with an increased signal on MRI, a bony impingement would be suggested and its physical presence may predispose to recurrent symptoms. Observing concurrent signal change in the tibia helps validate this opinion. In this case, surgical opinion will be important, to evaluate the risk of recurrence. An assessment of functional and mechanical instability of the ankle and how it may relate to posterior impingement signs is an important part of the management decision process.

Ankle Anterior Impingement

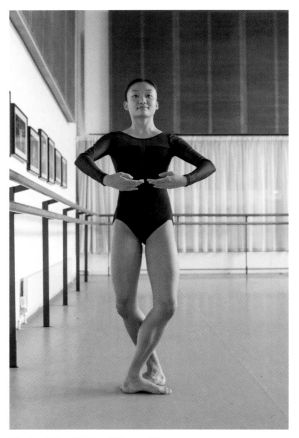

Photo 104   Plié in fifth position.

Similarly, due to the extreme ranges, anterior impingements during plié positions are prevalent in dancers. These may be anterior or anterior lateral in nature. Anterior impingement may relate to bony change and osteophytic lipping noted in the tibia. Anterior lateral impingements often relate to biomechanical adjustments causing overloading of soft tissue within the talocrural joint. Examination of the biomechanics of the plié movement (dorsiflexion in a weight-bearing posture) is important as part of the assessment. There is a natural medial obliquity through the ankle joint into dorsiflexion. In certain conditions, this is exaggerated and creates an impingement in the lateral aspect of the joint. This can be further assessed on a non-weight-bearing assessment of fibular translation. Typically, the fibula will translate cephalically and slightly laterally in dorsiflexion. A comparison of both ankles will help establish if this movement is being blocked due to the fibula, resulting in the ankle deviating and creating a greater medial shift through the talocrural joint.

Foot

The pattern of movement can be associated with a stiff subtalar joint and can also be responsible for increased mobility through the tarsometatarsal joint. The subtalar joint has a role in posture, via slight adjustments in inversion and eversion in the hindfoot. When the subtalar joint stiffens, the result is a compensatory adjustment of inversion and eversion movement through the midfoot. This may create increased loading through the medial structures of the midfoot, most importantly the navicular. Additionally, it may be responsible for increasing the load through the first metatarsolphalangeal joint (MTPJ). In dancers with a hallux valgus, this may present in the case of an aggravation of the condition. It may also result in pain through the first ray of the plantar fascia.

The forefoot is potentially susceptible to a greater prevalence of injury in dance than in many sports. Dancers are exposed to risk by the absence of supportive footwear, coupled with the loading demands and challenging postures used in dance. To reduce this, it is key to focus on the intrinsic risk inherent in the foot. This requires an appreciation of the role of the intrinsic layers of muscles supporting the region, as they are the primary support for the arches of the foot. It is essential for a healthcare practitioner working in dance to consider the intrinsic muscles of the first toe, which include the flexor hallucis brevis, adductor hallucis and abductor hallucis. The relationship between these key intrinsic muscles and the sesamoids is also an important consideration, with the medial aspect of the flexor hallucis brevis and abductor hallucis attaching to the medial sesamoid, and the lateral aspect of flexor hallucis brevis and adductor hallucis attaching to the lateral sesamoid. Development of a hallux valgus deformity is more noted in female dancers and may be associated with pointe work, when dancers fail to control this highly pressured position. The decision to move a young dancer to pointe work needs careful consideration and a confidence there is enough strength through the feet and legs to support it.

The nature of loading through the midfoot may increase the risk of developing several challenging pathologies. The presence of a Morton's toe, an elongated second metatarsal, can increase the risk of a stress reaction or fracture of the second metatarsal for dancers required to go en pointe. They would typically weight-bear through the first and second toe but, due to the increased length of the second toe, that joint becomes a focal point for loading. Similarly, dancers looking to offload their medial midfoot can inadvertently load their lateral midfoot. Stress responses in the lateral cuneiform have been reported in ballet dancers. The role of the cuboid bone in dancers is often a topic of discussion, with some suggesting that it can sublux and create symptoms. Given the shape and position of the bone, this seems unlikely, but its role in lateral midfoot biomechanics is important and comparisons to the unaffected foot regarding mobility are key to understanding its role in symptoms in a dancer's foot. With repeated demi-pointe work, metatarsolphalangeal synovitis is possible in dance. The presence of a V sign created by the toes confirms irritation here. Offloading, with NSAIDs, may alleviate symptoms. If this is unsuccessful, a local steroid injection can be a more powerful anti-inflammatory option. The rehabilitation programme needs to incorporate a correction of abnormal mechanics, alongside developing appropriate control of the foot in the demi-pointe position and calf capacity.

Although their prevalence is low, Morton's neuromas have been reported in ballet dancers. Professional ballet dancers' pointe shoes are custom made. Because of the aesthetic requirement in ballet, they are typically as narrow as they can be, which may increase the risk of developing a neuroma at the point where the metatarsals are pushed together while dancing. The challenge to healthcare teams is to determine the clinical significance of a neuroma. There is an ever-increasing opportunity to utilize radiology in modern sports medicine. It is possible up to 20 per cent of scans may demonstrate a neuroma, and it is also possible to observe a Mulders click on ultrasound, but neither of these findings will necessarily have any clinical relevance. An assessment of each patient's own symptoms is critical in interpreting the relevance of the neuroma. If a dancer presents with a clinically significant Morton's neuroma, it is worth looking at their shoes, as well as establishing whether their current production requires the shoes to be dyed, as this will affect the elastic properties of the shoe fabric.

The arches of the foot are further supported through the fibrous plantar fascia. It originates at the calcaneus and splits to attach to the five metatarsophalangeal joints. Heel pain in dancers is not uncommon. However, it is important to differentiate between potential sources. In addition to plantar fasciitis, heel fat pad bruising needs to be considered. The heel fat pad is a multi-chamber shock absorber that can easily be the recipient of traumatic impact during jumps. Patients with fat pad irritation tend to present with greater pain in the morning and find it persists through the day. Those with plantar fasciitis also present with increased pain in the morning, but may find that the area 'warms up' as the day goes on. Symptoms may be reduced with more (lower-level) activity but aggravated with increased loading or activity.

Management of heel pain associated with fat pad bruising entails reduced loading. Plantar fasciitis can be managed by support strapping in the early stages and by biomechanical corrections. There appears a high prevalence of reduced subtalar joint mobility in patients with plantar fasciitis but this responds well to manual therapy. Developing research also suggests a potential benefit from shockwave therapy in the management of this condition.

Ankle and Foot Fractures

Fractures of the ankle and foot have been reported in dance, including avulsion fractures of the lateral malleoli and fifth metatarsal associated with inversion injuries. Malleoli fractures are rare in dance, but they seem to be more common in contemporary dance, which may present more challenging choreography, with floor work sometimes combined with aerial work. Classification of such fractures uses the Danis-Webber Type system:

- A: below the joint line;
- B: level with the joint line;
- C: above the joint line.

A Webber Type A fracture is a simple fracture that can be managed according to pain and may not require any immobilization or treatment, other than an ankle support. A Webber Type B fracture needs to be investigated further, to establish whether it is stable. If no displacement is seen in weight-bearing x-rays, the fracture can be managed conservatively. Traditional management is usually 6 weeks of immobilization with partial weight-bearing started between week 3 and 4, depending on the extent of the fracture, the healing and the pain. However, a recent study (2019), published in the *British Medical Journal* by Kortekangas et.al., demonstrated no inferior results with 3 weeks of immobilization versus 6 weeks in Type B stable fractures. The benefit of a shorter immobilization period is that it may reduce the potential negative impacts of immobilization, such as muscle wasting and joint stiffness.

A Webber Type C fracture also requires further investigation, to establish whether it is stable.

Unstable Type B and C fractures require a surgical opinion. Fracture dislocations require surgical stabilization as well as an exploration of the talus, to establish the extent of damage to the chondral surface.

The forces needed to result in a Maisonneuve fracture following syndesmotic rupture are rare, but this needs to be part of the acute assessment of a dancer following high-velocity inversion. Additionally, spiral fractures of the fifth metatarsal are sometimes noted. Typically, treatment for a spiral fracture of the fifth may entail relative unloaded rest but, in the case of a Jones fracture, a surgical opinion needs to be sought. Due to the repeated loading and extremes of movement through the talocrural joint, awareness of osteochondral defects to the talar dome need to be considered in dancers who report pain in loaded plié positions.

Twisting movements in dance may have a significant impact on the midfoot. Although their prevalence is low, there is a high index of suspicion of lisfranc injuries with midfoot sprains. The stability of the second metatarsal is influenced by the three bands of the lisfranc ligaments. MRI is sensitive in establishing whether there has been damage to the ligaments. If a high signal is seen with the second metatarsal and medial cuneiform, this needs to be followed up with comparative AP and oblique weight-bearing x-ray (stork views), to establish if there is any lateral migration of the second metatarsal. It may also help confirm if an avulsion of the ligament has occurred. Management of a lisfranc injury is dependent on the grading. Like all sprains, it can range from a mild injury, which should respond to initial POLICE (Protect, Optimal Loading, Ice, Compression, Elevation) management, followed by a graded return to dance, to more severe sprains that require a period of immobilization to support the damaged ligament. Any evidence of instability as noted through the weight-bearing x-rays will warrant a surgical opinion.

Fractures of the calcaneus in dance are typically caused by high axial loading from the talus into the calcaneus in jumping, but can also include the anterior process of the calcaneus following plantar flexion and inversion injuries. Calcaneal fractures in dance are usually managed conservatively, with the exception of displaced fractures of the sustentaculum tali, posterior avulsion fractures or significant fractures. Similarly, fractures of the talus are unusual – typically sustained in a fall from height – but, given the complications associated with them due to blood supply and risk of avascular necrosis, need close attention and investigation. Management can be conservative or surgical.

Tendon Pathology of the Ankle and Foot

The lateral aspect of the ankle and foot can see adaptive changes such as tendinosis within the peroneal tendons, particularly associated with dancers with chronic ankle instability. A tendon loading programme is recommended in this case, with concentration on developing greater ankle stability, along with support from higher up the movement chain, including the hip. Peroneal dislocations and subluxations are associated with traumatic episodes in younger athletes and dancers, normally through dorsiflexion of an inverted foot. Non-traumatic episodes also need to be considered

in dance, with repeated trauma to the supporting retinaculum a potential risk to stability of the tendon region, particular if it is in the presence of a shallow fibular groove. Management of a subluxing peroneal tendon ranges from a period of immobilization to surgical repair of the peroneal retinaculum, with possible deepening of the fibula groove. With lateral ankle and lower leg pain, there is the potential of split tears. These tend to have a poor prognosis if managed conservatively and may require surgical intervention.

Achilles tendinopathy can be a challenging condition to manage in athletic populations. Research has suggested that eccentric loading of gastrocnemius and soleus can improve and manage symptoms. The high volume of gastrocnemius and soleus loading already seen in the typical day of a dancer may be the reason why there is a low prevalence when compared with other jumping sports. When tendinopathy is identified in a dancer, it is important to assess his or her plantar flexion capacity. When it has been established, employing an eccentric-biased loaded heel raise (straight and bent knee) programme can be very successful. It is important

Table 40   Achilles tendinopathy programme.

Tendinopathy session	Time (sec)	Reps	Sets
Inhibition			
Foam roller releases -- quads, hams, gluts and calf	20–60		
Neuromuscular facilitation – isometric			
Glut med/max isometric holds in flex and ext	8	8	2
Isometric ankle plantar flexion holds	45–60	4	2
Posterior fibular glides with resistance band and small knee bend/plié	NA		
Isolate/strengthen			
Eccentrics			
Eccentric heel rises (straight leg) (twice daily – progress to 3×)	NA	15	3
Eccentric heel rises (bent leg) (twice daily – progress to 3×)	NA	15	3
Hip eccentric external rotations	NA	15	3
Functional integration			
Hop and holds on to 1 leg (controlled landing through foot/knee/hip)		12–15	3–4
Heel drop rebound 'beats' (in turn-out)		12–15	3–4
Jump box landing drill (controlled landing through foot/knee/hip)		12–15	3–4
Jump box take-off drill (controlled landing through foot/knee/hip)		12–15	3–4

to use this period to explore and change any biomechanical anomalies. The presence of reduced subtalar mobility, coupled with increased plantar fascia tension, suggests a more global mechanical loading issue, where the impact of control of centre of gravity/pressure through effective postural control can be employed. Sometimes, a patient's level of pain will be high enough to restrict their ability to undertake a loading programme. In these cases, the use of high-volume tendon-stripping injections (typically saline) can be effective to reduce the pain and allow rehabilitation to take place.

Table 41   Tibialis posterior rehabilitation programme.

Exercise and progression	Description: session A (perform 2× day 3× week	Progressive overload		
		Reps per set	Sets	Rest between sets
1. Side-lying isometric hip extension		3–5/leg with 7sec hold	2	3sec between contract
2. Side-lying hip ext rotation		3–5/leg with 7sec hold	2	3secisometric between contract
3. Swiss ball straight-leg bridge (SL)	Feet on Swiss ball, lying flat on back	10–12	2	30sec
4. Swiss ball reverse bridge (SL)	Shoulders on Swiss ball	10–12	2	30sec
5. Side-lying leg lift (int rot)	5 sec hold – possibly add small ankle weight (2kg)	6–8	3	30sec
6. Side-lying leg lift (ext rot)	5 sec hold – possibly add small ankle weight (2kg)	6–8	3	30sec
7. 'Over a step' tib post drops	Emphasis on flattening and arching the medial longitudinal arch	6–8	3	30sec
8. Monster resistance band walks	Pressure through trail leg while maintaining medial longitudinal arch	10/direction	2	30sec
9. Heel rise with isometric tib post pull	Heel rise with theraband pulling at 45deg medially creating an isometric contraction of tib post	15–25	2–3	30sec

Adaptive changes to the flexor hallucis longus and tibialis posterior appear more prevalent in dancers than in other sporting populations. Because of its role in initiating plantar flexion and then stabilizing the midfoot in the plantar flexed position, the tibialis posterior is at risk of overuse injury in dance, with excessive rising, pointe and demi-pointe work. As with Achilles management, loading programmes are useful in the management of tibialis posterior tendinopathy, but success will also depend on identifying the causation. A thorough biomechanical assessment is essential, including evaluations further up the movement chain, to the hip and sacroiliac joint. Failure to control turn-out will result in 'navicular drop' and excessive loading of the tibialis posterior eccentrically, as it works to maintain medial longitudinal arch posture. Improvements in femoral anteversion control may offset the loading to tibialis posterior significantly. An additional consequence of this can be increased loading of the first metatarsolphalangeal joint (MTPJ). Coupled with a dancer's use of turn-out, this can increase loading of the medial sesamoid and result in sesamoid pathology, including sesamoiditis, stress responses and fractures. The position of the medial sesamoid is influenced by the angle of the phalanges. In the case of a hallux valgus deformity, the medial sesamoid can find itself in a more load-bearing position, greatly increasing its vulnerability to injury.

Rehabilitation and conditioning in the case of tibialis posterior tendinopathy involves biomechanical correction and eccentric control into femoral anteversion. Additionally, applying eccentric loading through the plantar flexion movement is important in improving the tensile loading capacity of the tendon. If higher loading strategies are employed, offload days should be allowed as part of the recovery. These do, however, need to be balanced with creating a suitable chronic training load, in order to build a robust capacity to enable the dancer to tolerate the typical work in dance. An example of an early- to middle-stage programme is shown in Table 41.

Flexor hallucis longus tendinopathy and split tears have been described in ballet. Dancers use their first toe to help accentuate the pointing of the foot as well as to help stabilize their position while en pointe, and this increases the loading of this muscle. Split tears can be difficult to detect, as MRI and even ultrasound are not always sensitive to such small changes. Clinical history and response to treatment and rehabilitation programmes occasionally provide the additional evidence needed to pursue this area further.

There are descriptions in sports medicine literature of intersection syndrome in the wrist, with the crossing-over and irritation of the abductor pollicis longus and extensor pollicis brevis. While it is infrequent, intersection syndrome may need to be considered in dancers, at the master knot of Henry in the foot, where the tendon of flexor digitorum longus passes obliquely over flexor hallucis longus, around the region of the navicular. The dancer may present with plantar midfoot pain, which may have a variety of sources, from local inflammatory changes to fibrosis of the knot. In the case of inflammatory changes, management with offloading and anti-inflammatories may suffice. In the case of fibrosis, a surgical opinion may be needed.

Plantar Plate Injuries

Plantar plate injuries can occur to the metatarsal phalangeal joint (MTPJ) of the first or the lesser toes. The plantar plate is a complex area, with a number of structures under the metatarsal phalangeal joint. The region comprises cartilaginous plate that originates from a thin synovial attachment in continuity with the metatarsal metaphysis periosteum. It inserts via a firm fibrocartilaginous attachment into the base of the proximal phalanx. It has additional support via the distil plantar fascia, accessory collateral ligament, transverse metatarsal ligament, interosseous tendons and fibrous sheath of flexor tendons. The role of the plantar plate is to stabilize and cushion the MTPJ during weight-bearing. It does this through passive extension during gait or demi-pointe positions. The fat pad of the metatarsal heads moves over the plantar plate to cover the metatarsal head and act as a shock absorber. Furthermore, it resists tensile loading in a longitudinal direction and supports the windlass mechanism via the contribution of the plantar fascia. It serves as an attachment for inter-metatarsal and collateral ligaments and resists varus and valgus strain and dorsal instability.

Damage in this area is likely to have occurred as the result of either attenuation of the structure over time due to abnormal biomechanics and load, or traumatic loading, or a combination of the two. Management of plantar plate injuries can be conservative or surgical, largely depending on the degree of damage and stability. The modified Lachmanns test for MTPJ stability, called the Hamilton-Thompson MTPJ drawer test, can be used to classify stability. Classification ranges from G0 (stable) through to G4 (a dislocated joint). Irrespec-

tive of whether the management route is surgical or conservative, correction of biomechanics is critical. Identifying movement competency around triple flexion movements, such as a squat position and plié, and relevé, are important due to the role of the plantar plate in cushioning and stabilizing the MTPJ. By creating optimal posterior chain control, it is possible to move the centre of pressure and reduce load through the MTPJs and plantar plate. Furthermore, considering its role in resisting tensile loading in the longitudinal direction and supporting the windlass mechanism via its contribution of plantar fascia, developing control of femoral anteversion and navicular drop through eccentric control of the hip external rotators, tibialis posterior and the intrinsic muscles of the foot is critical.

CONCLUSION

Whether they can be considered to be artists or athletes, what dancers do is truly exceptional. Through their story-telling, they are able to evoke emotions, and the fluidity of movement they demonstrate sets them apart from other occupational athletes. Scientists cannot fail to appreciate the functional outputs achieved by a dancer, despite physiological variables such as strength and fitness that are not equivalent to those seen in high-performance sports.

In comparison with high-performance sport, where commercialization and the influx of television money and funding have allowed better support structures that have fuelled research and investment in medical care, dance is still a relatively poorly supported discipline. The purpose of this book is to look at the challenges faced in providing a suitable level of care for dancers, highlighting the way in which dance may fit within the current aetiological models of injury and how that information may be used to help reduce the impact of injury in dance. Clearly, well-structured injury data collection, with examples from clinicians working directly in dance, facilitates the monitoring of injury in dance, and informs healthcare practitioners about its impact.

The role of complementary conditioning in dance has become important. While dance has traditionally relied on a very functionally biased approach to training, the advancement in knowledge in sports science and, as part of that, dance medicine, has demonstrated where additional conditioning can support and enhance performance capacity as well as reduce the risk of injury. Strength, power and muscle endurance can play a key role in supporting a dancer.

The development of injury prevention programmes in dance is built out of the aetiological models and targets aspects of intrinsic, extrinsic and modifiable risk. Early-stage injury management follows the same pattern as in sport, with the POLICE (Protect, Optimal Loading, Ice, Compression, Elevation) procedure, and recent developments around optimal loading are a key inclusion to the traditional ICE and PRICE (Protection, Rest, Ice, Compression, Elevation) protocols.

A dysfunctional biomechanical cycle in a dancer can influence injury presentations and the healthcare practitioner must be aware of the potential impact of this if success in patient management and outcomes is to be achieved. The Hybrid Intervention Model is a means by which a suitable rehabilitation programme for a dancer can be structured. The model builds on key limiting factors in injury, namely pain/structural damage, causation or movement weakness, and the outcomes required. It then relates these to the relative ratios of the three components of the rehabilitation programme – neuromuscular

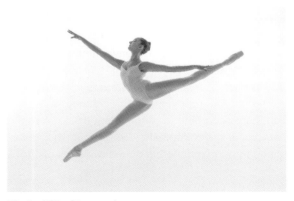

Photo 105 Sissonné. KIRSTY WALKER

facilitation, segmental deficit training and functional integration training – and how they may alter as a dancer progresses through the various stages of the injury cycle, from early or acute injury to end stage. As part of the segmental deficit training component, blood flow restriction may be a way of addressing strength deficits while still using low loads. Exit criteria and testing for a return to dance are vital, along with a long-term rehabilitation programme.

The anatomy and biomechanics of the various regions of the body relate in very specific ways to dance and its injuries. Some outcomes are potentially severe, and there is a growing understanding in the sports medicine community about the need to have robust management strategies in place. One example is concussion, which, despite it having a relatively low incidence compared with contact sports, must be managed correctly. There are also strategies that focus on injuries that have a higher incidence in dance, such as those that affect the foot and ankle region, and lateral ligament sprains or posterior impingements.

There are a number of factors that clinicians working in dance will need to be aware of, particularly when working with adolescent and child dancers. The impact of growth on injury is an area currently being explored in dance, as it has been in sport. The impact of repetitive loading on immature joints and bone is an important consideration. Certain paediatric conditions, such as Osgood-Schlatter or Severs disease, or even a developing scoliosis, need specialist attention if their impact in later life is to be reduced. Sports scientists have identified key areas where an adolescent athlete needs to develop the physiological characteristics that will be required in a high-performance sports environment. A typical long-term athlete development timeline will look at windows of trainability in areas such as speed, strength, skill or movement competency, and position them according to various periods in the young participant's development. These may be determined through monitoring of peak velocity changes (growth spurts), for example. In dance, this can be expanded to identify, for example, the age at which it would be appropriate to move on to higher-risk activities, like starting pointe work. As in sport, the use of biological ages is often inappropriate as there can be a notable disparity between biological and maturation age in children. Decision-making needs to take both into account, alongside an adequate assessment of the strength and technical capacity of the whole lower-leg kinetic chain. Undertaking pointe work too soon may lead to development of hallux valgus as a senior dancer.

Another major consideration when dealing with a dancer is the psychological impact of injury and the pressure to fulfil performance requirements. There is growing research showing that certain personality types are drawn to competitive and high-performance environments. Clinicians have a duty of care to be mindful of the risk of tipping into areas that affect dancer's mental health and wellbeing. Professional dancers often start their pathway to a career in dance from a very early age, with many entering vocational school training at 11. This commitment can result in anxiety when facing any injury, and this may be particularly severe if it is potentially career-threatening. Understanding such issues is an important part of the overall management of dancers and needs to be taken into account when planning a rehabilitation programme. The dancer must be psychologically ready to return to dance as well as physically ready. The psychological readiness is relevant through all stages of the rehabilitation process and the use of mental imagery as part of rehabilitation has been successful in dance.

There is a growing national agenda of 'dance for health', with dance offering a means to support the physical and mental health of the general population. It is an excellent form of exercise, particularly for those individuals who may not have enjoyed sport, so it is vitally important for dance medicine to continue to develop the knowledge to support every participant. Let's 'Keep Dancing'!

BIBLIOGRAPHY

Allen, N., Neville, A., Brooks, J., Koutedakis, Y. & Wyon, M. (2012). Ballet injuries: injury incidence and severity over one year. J Orthop Sports Phys Ther Sep;**42**(9), pp.781–90

Allen, N., Neville, A., Brooks, J., Koutedakis, Y. & Wyon, M. (2013). The Effect of a Comprehensive Injury Audit Programme on Injury Incidence in Ballet: A 3-Year Prospective Study Clin J Sport Med. 2013 Sep; **23**(5):373–8. doi: 10.1097/JSM.0b013e3182887f32

Allen, N. & Williams, W. (2014). Musculoskeletal Injuries in Dance: A Systematic Review DOI: 10.4172/2329–9096.1000252

Allen, N. & Wyon, M. (2008). Dance Medicine: Athlete or Artist. *SportEx Medicine*, **35**, pp.6–9

Andrews, J., Guyatt, G., Oxman, A., Alderson, P. et al. (2013). GRADE guidelines: 14. Going from evidence to recommendations: the significance and presentation of recommendations. *Journal of Clinical Epidemiology.* **66**(7), pp.719–725

Angioi, M., Twitchett, E., Metsios, G., Koutedakis, Y. & Wyon, M. (2009). Association between selected physical fitness parameters and aesthetic competence in contemporary dance. *Journal of Dance Medicine and Science*, **13**(4), pp.115–123

AQA (2009) Awarding body for A-levels, GCSEs and other exams. Available at aqa.org.uk/index.php

Arthur, W., Bennet, W., Stanush, P. & McNelly, T. (1998). Factors that influence skill decay and retention: A quantitative review and analysis. *Human Performance*, **11**(1), pp.57–101

The Arts Council (2009). Dance Mapping: a window on dance. Available at artscouncil.org.uk/media/uploads/publications/dance_mapping_full_report.pdf

Asplund, C. & Ross, M. (2010). Core stability and bicycling. *Current Sports Medicine Reports*, **9**(3), pp.155–160

Augustsson, S., Augustsson, J., Thomée, R. & Svantesson, U. (2006). Injuries and preventive actions in elite Swedish volleyball. *Scandinavian Journal of Medicine and Science in Sports*, **16**(6), pp.433–440

Bahr, R. (2009). No injuries, but plenty of pain? On the methodology for recording overuse symptoms in sports. *British Journal of Sports Medicine*, **43**(13), pp.966–972

Bahr, R. & Holme, I. (2003). Risk factors for sports injuries – a methodological approach. *British Journal of Sports Medicine*, **37**(5), pp.384–392

Bahr, R. & Krosshaug, T. (2005). Understanding injury mechanisms: a key component of preventing injuries in sport. [Review]. *British Journal of Sports Medicine*, **39**(6), pp.324–329

Balshem, H., Helfand, M., Schünemann, H., Oxman, A., Kunz, R., Brozek, J., Vist, G., Falck-Ytter, Y., Meerpohl, J., Norris, S. & Guyatt, G. (2011) GRADE guidelines: 3. Rating the quality of evidence. *Journal of Clinical Epidemiology.* **64**(4), pp.401–406

Banton, R. (2012). *The Journal of the Spinal Research Foundation* **7**(2012), pp.12–20

Batt, M. E., Jaques, R. & Stone, M. (2004). Preparticipation Examination (Screening): Practical Issues as Determined by Sport: A United Kingdom Perspective. *Clinical Journal of Sport Medicine*, **14**(3), pp.178–182

Batten, Taylor, Cook, Pizzari, & Charlton. (2010). Key musculoskeletal screening tests used in Australian Football have limited reliability. *Journal of Science and Medicine in Sport*, **12**, e167

Beales, D., O'Sullivan, Peter, & Briffa, N. (2009a). Motor Control Patterns During an Active Straight Leg Raise in Chronic Pelvic Girdle Pain Subjects. *Spine*, **34**, pp.861–870

Beales, D., O'Sullivan, Peter, & Briffa, N. (2009b). Motor Control Patterns During an Active Straight Leg Raise in Pain-Free Subjects. *Spine*, **34**, pp.E1-E8

Beattie, K. A., Bobba, R., Bayoumi, I., Chan, D., Schabort, I., Boulos, P. et al. (2008). Validation of the GALS musculoskeletal screening exam for use in primary care: a pilot study. *BMC Musculoskeletal Disorders*, **9**, 115, pp.1–8

Bennell, K., Tully, E. & Harvey, N. (1999). Does the toe-touch test predict hamstring injury in Australian rules footballers? *Australian Journal of Physiotherapy*, **45**(2), pp.103–109

Bennell, K. L., Khan, K. M., Matthews, B. L. & Singleton, C. (2001). Changes in hip and ankle range of motion and hip muscle strength in 8–11 year old novice female ballet dancers and controls: a 12 month follow up study. *British Journal of Sports Medicine*, **35**(1), pp.54–59

Bennett, J. E., Reinking, M. F., Pluemer, B., Pentel, A., Seaton, M. & Killian, C. (2001). Factors contributing to the development of medial tibial stress syndrome in high school runners. *Journal of Orthopaedic and Sports Physical Therapy*, **31**(9), pp.504–510

Boardley, I. Allen, N. et al. (2015). Nutritional, medicinal, and performance enhancing supplementation in dance. *Performance Enhancement and Health* **4**(1)

Bowling, A. (1989). Injuries to dancers: prevalence, treatment, and perceptions of causes. *British Medical Journal (Clinical Research Ed.)*, **298**(6675), pp.731–734

Bradley, P. S. & Portas, M. D. (2007). The relationship between preseason range motion and muscle strain injury in elite soccer players. *Journal of Strength and Conditioning Research*, **21**(4), pp.1155–1159

Briggs, J., McCormack, M., Hakim, A. J., & Grahame, R. (2009). Injury and joint hypermobility syndrome in ballet dancers – a 5-year follow-up. *Rheumatology*, **48**(12), pp.1613–1614

Briggs, M. Givens, D. Best, T. & Chaudhari, A. (2013). Lumbopelvic neuromuscular training and injury rehabilitation: a systematic review. *Clinical Journal of Sport Medicine*, **23** pp.160–171

Brinson, P. & Dick, F. (1996). Fit to dance? The report of the national inquiry into dancers' health and injury. London: Calouste Gulbenkian Foundation

British Association of Sports and Exercise Medicine. (2010). Aims – Activities. Available from http://www.basem.co.uk/aims-activities/201/false/39/201

Bronner, S. & Brownstein, B. (1997). Profile of dance injuries in a Broadway show: a discussion of issue in dance medicine epidemiology. *Journal of Orthopaedic and Sports Physical Therapy*, **26**(2), pp.87–94

Bronner, S., Ojofeitimi, S. & Mayers, L. (2006). Comprehensive surveillance of dance injuries: a proposal for uniform reporting guidelines for professional companies. *Journal of Dance Medicine and Science*, **10**(3–4), pp.69–80

Bronner, S., Ojofeitimi, S. & Rose, D. (2003). Injuries in a modern dance company. Effect of comprehensive management on injury incidence and time loss. *American Journal of Sports Medicine*, **31**(3), pp.365–373

Brooks, J. H., Fuller, C. W., Kemp, S.P., Reddin, D. B. (2005). A prospective study of injuries and training amongst the England 2003 Rugby World Cup squad. *British Journal of Sports Medicine*, **39**(5), pp.288–293

Brooks, J. H. M., & Fuller, C. W. (2006). The Influence of Methodological Issues on the Results and Conclusions from Epidemiological Studies of Sports Injuries: Illustrative Examples. *Sports Medicine*, **36**(6), pp.459–472

Brooks, J. H. M., Fuller, C. W., Kemp, S. P. T. & Reddin, D. B. (2005a). Epidemiology of injuries in English professional rugby union: part 1 match injuries. *British Journal of Sports Medicine*, **39**(10), pp.757–766

Brooks, J. H. M., Fuller, C. W., Kemp, S. P. T. & Reddin, D. B. (2005b). Epidemiology of injuries in English professional rugby union: part 2 training Injuries. *British Journal of Sports Medicine*, **39**(10), pp.767–775

Brozek, J., Akl, E., Alonso-Coello, P. et al. for the GRADE Working Group (2009). Grading quality of evidence and strength of recommendations in clinical practice guidelines. Part 1 of 3. An overview of the GRADE approach and grading quality of evidence about interventions. *Allergy*, **64**: pp.669–677

Brozek, J. Akl, E. Jaeschke, R. et al. for the GRADE Working Group (2009). Grading quality of evidence and strength of recommendations in clinical practice guidelines. Part 2 of 3. The GRADE approach to grading quality of evidence about diagnostic tests and strategies. *Allergy*, **64**: pp.1109–1116

Brozek, J. Akl, E. Compalati, E. et al. for the GRADE Working Group (2011). Grading quality of evidence and strength of recommendations in clinical practice guidelines. Part 3 of 3. The GRADE approach to developing recommendations. *Allergy*, **66**: pp.588–595

Brunetti, M. Shemilt, I. Pregno, S. Vale, L. et al. (2013) GRADE guidelines: 10. Considering resource use and rating the quality of economic evidence. *Journal of Clinical Epidemiology*, **66**,2: pp.40–150

Brushoj, C. Larsen, K. Albrecht-Beste, E. Bachmann Nielsen, M. Loye, F. & Homlich, P.(2008). Prevention of overuse injuries by a concurrent exercise programme in subjects exposed to an increase in training overload: A randomized controlled trial of 1020 Army recruits. *American Journal of Sports Medicine*, **36**, pp.663–672

Chorbra, R., Chorbra, D., Bouillon, L., Overmyer, C. & Landis, J. (2010). Use of a functional movement screening tool to determine injury risk female collegiate athletes. *North American Journal of Sports Physical Therapy*, **5**, 2: 47–54

Chmelar, R., Fitt, B., Schultz, R., Ruhling, O. & Zupan, M. (1987). A survey of health, training and injuries in different levels and styles of dancers. *Medical Problems of Performing Artists*, **2**(2), pp.61–66

Choi, B. K. L., Verbeek, J. H., Tam, W. W. S. & Jiang, J. Y. Exercises for prevention of recurrences of low-back pain. *Cochrane Database of Systematic Reviews 2010*, Issue **1**. Art. No.: CD006555. DOI: 10.1002/14651858.CD006555.pub2

Clippinger, K. S. (2005) 'Biomechanical Considerations in Turnout.' In Solomon, Ruth (ed.), *Preventing Dance Injuries*. 2nd ed, Champaign, Ill., *Human Kinetics*, 2005, pp.109;135–150.

Comerford, M. J. (2006). Screening to identify injury and performance risk: movement control testing – the missing piece of the puzzle. *SportEX Medicine* **29**, pp.1–26

Cook, E., Burton, L., & Hogenboom, B. (2006a). The use of fundamental movements as an assessment of function – Part 1. *North American Journal of Sports Physical Therapy*, **1**, pp.62–72

Cook, E., Burton, L., & Hogenboom, B. (2006b). The use of fundamental movements as an assessment of function – Part 2. *North American Journal of Sports Physical Therapy*, **1**, pp.132–139

Coplan, J. (2002) Ballet dancers' turnout and its relationship to self-reported injury. *Orthopaedic and Sports Physical Therapy*, **32**, pp.11, 579–584

Coughlan, G. & Caulfield, B. (2007). A 4-week neuromuscular training program and gait patterns at the ankle joint. *Journal of Athletic Training*, **42**(1);51–59

Craig, P. (2008) Developing and evaluating complex interventions: the new Medical Research Council guidance. *British Medical Journal* vol. **337** pp.1655–1680

Cusi, M. F., Paradigm for assessment and treatment of SIJ mechanical dysfunction, *Journal of Bodywork & Movement Therapies* (2010), doi: 10.1016/j.jbmt.2009.12.004

Dahlstrom, M., Inasio, J., Jansson, E. & Kaijser, L.(1996) Physical fitness and physical effort in dancers: a comparison of four major dance styles. *Impulse*, **4**: pp 193–209

Dahm, P. & Djulbegovic, B. (2011) The Australian FORM approach to guideline development: the quest for the perfect system. *BMC Medical Research Methodology*, **11**:17

DanceUK (2010). Dance UK – The National Voice For Dance – Dance Facts and Stats. Available at http://www.danceuk.org/metadot/index.pl?iid=25043&isa=Category

Dankaerts, W., O'Sullivan, P., Burnett, A. & Straker, L. (2006). Differences in sitting postures are associated with nonspecific chronic low back pain disorders when patients are subclassified. *Spine*, **31** (6), pp.698–704

de Loes, M. (1997). Exposure data. Why are they needed. *Sports Medicine*, **24**(3), pp.172–175

Dennis, Finch, Elliot & Farhart (2008). The reliability of musculoskeletal screening tests used in cricket. *Physical Therapy in Sport*, **9**, pp.25–33

Dennis, A. J., Finch, C. F., McIntosh, A. S. & Elliott, B. C. (2008). Use of field-based tests to identify risk factors for injury to fast bowlers in cricket. *British Journal of Sports Medicine*, **42**(6), pp.477–482

De Vries, J. S., Krips, R., Sierevelt, I. N. et al. (2011). Interventions for treating chronic ankle instability. *Cochrane Database of Systematic Reviews*. **8**:CD004124

Department of Health. (2009). Be Active Be Healthy. Available at http://www.dh.gov.uk/prod_consum_dh/groups/dh_digitalassets/documents/digitalasset/dh_094359.pdf

Drawer, S. & Fuller, C. W. (2001). Propensity for osteoarthritis and lower limb joint pain in retired professional soccer players... including commentary by Waddington I. *British Journal of Sports Medicine*, **35**(6), pp.402–408

Elwood, J. (1988). Causal relationship in medicine. A practical system for critical appraisal. Oxford University Press

Emery, C. Meeuwisse, W. (2007). The effectiveness of a neuromuscular prevention strategy to reduce injuries in youth soccer: a cluster-randomised control trial. *British Journal of Sports Medicine*, **44**(8), pp.555–562

Engebretsen, L. & Bahr, R. (2005). An ounce of prevention? *British Journal of Sports Medicine*, **39**(6), pp.312–313

Evans, R. W., Evans, R. I. & Carvajal, S. (1996). Survey of injuries among Broadway performers: Types of injuries, treatments and perceptions of performers. *Medical Problems of Performing Artists*, **11**(1), pp.15–19

Federici, A., Bellagamba, S., Rocchi, M. (2005). Does dance-based training improve balance in adult and young subjects? A pilot randomized control trial. *Aging clinical and experimental research*, **17**, (5), pp.385–389

Fentem, P. H. (1994). ABC of Sports Medicine: Benefits of exercise in health and disease. *British Medical Journal*, **308**(6939), pp.291–1295

Finch, C. F. (1997). An overview of some definitional issues for sports injury surveillance. *Sports Medicine*, **24**(3), pp.57–163

Fuller, C. W., Bahr, R., Dick, R. W. & Meeuwisse, W. H. (2007a). A framework for recording recurrences, reinjuries, and exacerbations in injury surveillance. *Clinical Journal of Sport Medicine*, **17**(3), pp.97–200

Fuller, C. and Drawer, S. (2004). The application of risk management in sport. *Sports Medicine*, **34**(6), pp.49–356

Fuller, C. W., Ekstrand, J., Junge, A., Andersen, T. E., Bahr, R., Dvorak, J. et al. (2006). Consensus statement on injury definitions and data collection procedures in studies of football (soccer) injuries. Scandinavian *Journal of Medicine & Science in Sports*, **16**(2), pp.83–92

Fuller, C. W., Molloy, M. G., Bagate, C., Bahr, R., Brooks, J. H. M., Donson, H. et al. (2007b). Consensus statement on injury definitions and data collection procedures for studies of injuries in rugby union. *Clinical Journal of Sport Medicine: Official Journal of The Canadian Academy Of Sport Medicine*, **17**(3), pp.177–181

Fuller, C. W., Ojelade, E. O. & Taylor, A. (2007c). Preparticipation medical evaluation in professional sport in the UK: theory or practice? *British Journal of Sports Medicine*, **41**(12), pp.890–896

Fransen, M., McConnell, S. Exercise for osteoarthritis of the knee. (2008) *Cochrane Database of Systematic Reviews*. **4**: CD004376. DOI: 10.1002/14651858.CD004376.pub2

Fransen, M., McConnell, S., Hernandez-Molina, G. & Reichenbach, S. (2009). Exercise for osteoarthritis of the hip. *Cochrane Database of Systematic Reviews*. **3**: CD007912. DOI: 10.1002/14651858.CD007912

Gabbe, B. J., Bennell, K. L., Wajswelner, H. & Finch, C. F. (2004). Reliability of common lower extremity musculoskeletal screening tests. *Physical Therapy in Sport*, **5**(2), 90–97

Gabbe, B. J., Finch, C. F., Bennell, K. L. & Wajswelner, H. (2003). How valid is a self-reported 12 month sports injury history? *British Journal of Sports Medicine*, **37**(6), pp.545–547

Gabbett, T. J. (2003). Incidence of injury in semi-professional rugby league players... including commentary by Phillips J. H. *British Journal of Sports Medicine*, **37**(1), pp.36–44

Gamboa, J. M., Roberts, L. A., Maring, J. & Fergus, A. (2008). Injury Patterns in Elite Preprofessional Ballet Dancers and the Utility of Screening Programs to Identify Risk Characteristics. *Journal of Orthopaedic and Sports Physical Therapy*, **38**(3), pp.126–136

Garrick, J. G. and Requa, R. K. (1993). Ballet injuries: an analysis of epidemiology and financial outcome. *American Journal of Sports Medicine*, **21**(4), pp.586–590

Gribble, P. A., Brigle, J., Pietrosimone, B. G., Pfile, K. R. & Webster, K. A. (2013) Intrarater reliability of the functional movement screen. *Journal of Strength Conditioning Research*, **27**(4), pp.978–981

Guyatt, G., Oxman, A., Akl, E., Kunz, R., Vist, G., Brozek, J., Norris, S., Falck-Ytter, Y., Glasziou, P., de Beer, H., Jaeschke, R., Rind, D., Meerpohl, J., Dahm, P. & Schünemann, H. (2011) GRADE guidelines: 1. Introduction – GRADE evidence profiles and summary of findings tables. *Journal of Clinical Epidemiology*. **64**, 4: pp.383–394

Guyatt, G., Oxman, A., Kunz, R., Atkins, D. et al. (April 2011) GRADE guidelines: 2. Framing the question and deciding on important outcomes. *Journal of Clinical Epidemiology*. **64**, 4: pp.395–400

Guyatt, G., Oxman, A., Vist, G., Kunz, R. et al. (April 2011) GRADE guidelines: 4. Rating the quality of evidence – study limitations (risk of bias). *Journal of Clinical Epidemiology*. **64**, 4: pp.407–415

Guyatt, G., Oxman, A., Montori, V., Vist, G. et al. (2011). GRADE guidelines: 5. Rating the quality of evidence – publication bias. *Journal of Clinical Epidemiology*. **64**, 12: pp.1277–1282

Guyatt, G., Oxman, A., Kunz, R., Brozek, J. et al. (2011) GRADE guidelines 6. Rating the quality of evidence – imprecision. *Journal of Clinical Epidemiology*. **64**, 12: pp.1283–1293

Guyatt, G., Oxman, A., Kunz, R., Woodcock, J. et al. (2011) GRADE guidelines: 7. Rating the quality of evidence – inconsistency. *Journal of Clinical Epidemiology*. **64**, 12: pp.1294–1302

Guyatt, G., Oxman, A., Kunz, R., Woodcock, J. et al. (2011). GRADE guidelines: 8. Rating the quality of evidence – indirectness. *Journal of Clinical Epidemiology*. **64**, 12: pp.1303–1310

Guyatt, G., Oxman, A., Sultan, S., Glasziou, P. et al. (2011) GRADE guidelines: 9. Rating up the quality of evidence. *Journal of Clinical Epidemiology*. **64**, 12: pp.1311–1316

Guyatt, G., Oxman, A., Sultan, S., Brozek, J. et al. (2013) GRADE guidelines: 11. Making an overall rating of confidence in effect estimates for a single outcome and for all outcomes. *Journal of Clinical Epidemiology*. **66**, 2: pp.151–157

Guyatt, G., Oxman, A., Santesso, N., Helfand, M. et al. (2013). GRADE guidelines: 12. Preparing summary of findings tables – binary outcomes. *Journal of Clinical Epidemiology*. **66**, 2: pp.158–172

Guyatt, G., Thorlund, K., Oxman, A., Walter, S. et al. (2013) GRADE guidelines: 13. Preparing summary of findings tables and evidence profiles- continuous outcomes. *Journal of Clinical Epidemiology*. **66**, 2: pp.173–183

Hakkinen, A., Makinen, H., Ylinen, J., Hannonen, P., Sokka, T., Neva, M., Kautiainen, H. & Kauppi, M. (2008). Stability of the upper neck during isometric neck exercises in rheumatoid arthritis patients with atlantoaxial disorders. *Scandinavian Journal of Rheumatology*, **37**(5), pp.343–347

Halbertsma, J. P. K., Göeken, L. N. H., Hoff, A. L., Groothoff, J. W., & Eisma, W. H. (2001). Extensibility and stiffness of the hamstring in patients with nonspecific low back pain. *Archives of Physical Medicine & Rehabilitation*, **82**(2), pp.232–238

Hamilton D, Aronsen P, Løken J, et al. (2006). Dance training intensity at 11–14 years is associated with femoral torsion in classical ballet dancers. *British Journal of Sports Medicine*, **40**, pp.299–303

Hans-Wilhelm Mueller-Wohlfahrt, Lutz Haensel, Kai Mithoefer, et al. Terminology and classification of muscle injuries in sport: The Munich Consensus Statement. *Br J Sports Med* 2012;0:1–9. doi:10.1136/bjsports–2012–091448

Hayen, A., Dennis, R. and Finch, C. (2007). Determining the intra- and inter-observer reliability of screening tools used in sports injury research. *Journal of Science and Medicine in Sport*, **10**(4), pp.201–210

Hayden, J., van Tulder, M. W., Malmivaara, A., & Koes, B. W. (2005) Exercise therapy for treatment of non-specific low back pain. *Cochrane Database of Systematic Reviews* 2005, Issue **3**. Art. No.: CD000335. DOI: 10.1002/14651858.CD000335. pub2

Heintjes, E. M., Berger, M., Bierma-Zeinstra, S. M. A., Bernsen, R. M. D., Verhaar, J. A. N. & Koes, B. W. (2003). Exercise therapy for patellofemoral pain syndrome. *Cochrane Database of Systematic Reviews*, Issue **4**. Art. No.: CD003472. DOI: 10.1002/14651858.CD003472

Herbert, R. D. & Gabriel, M. (2002). Effects of stretching before and after exercising on muscle soreness and risk of injury: systematic review. *British Medical Journal*, **325**(7362), pp.468–473

Herman, K., Barton, C., Malliaras, P. & Morrissey, D. (2012). The effectiveness of neuromuscular warm-up strategies, that require no additional equipment, for preventing lower limb injuries during sports participation: a systematic review. *BMC Medicine*, **10**:75

Hershman, E. (1984). The profile for prevention of musculoskeletal injury. *Clinics in Sports Medicine*, **3**(1), pp.65–84

Hewett, T., Ford, K. & Myer, G. (2006). Anterior cruciate ligament injuries in female athletes: Part 2, a meta-analysis of neuromuscular interventions aimed at injury prevention. *American Journal of Sports Medicine*, **3**4(3), pp.490–498

Higher Education Statistics Agency. (2009). Available at hesa.ac.uk

Hides, J., Jull, G. & Richardson, C. (2001). Long-term effects of specific stabilizing exercises for first episode low back pain. *Spine*, **26**(11), pp.243–248

Hincapie, C. A., Morton, E. J. & Cassidy, J. D. (2008). Musculoskeletal injuries and pain in dancers: a systematic review. *Archives of Physical Medicine and Rehabilitation*, **89**(9), pp.1819–1829

Hodges, P. & Moseley, G. (2003). Pain and motor control of the lumbo-pelvic region: Effect and possible mechanisms. *Journal of Electromyography and Kinesiology*, **4**, pp.361–370

Hodges, P. & Richardson, C. (1996). Inefficient muscular stabilization of the lumbar spine associated with low back pain: a motor control evaluation of transverse abdominis. *Spine*, **21**, pp.2640–2650

Hodgson-Phillips, L. (2000). Sports injury incidence. *British Journal of Sports Medicine*, **34**(2), pp.133–136

Hodgson, L., Gissane, C., Gabbett, T. & King, D. (2007). For Debate: consensus injury definitions in team sports should focus on encompassing all injuries. *Clinical Journal of Sport Medicine*, **17**(3), pp.188–191

Hopper, L. & Allen, N (2013) Dance floor mechanical properties and dancer injuries in a touring professional ballet company DOI: 10.1016/j.jsams.2013.04.013

Hopper, L. & Allen, N. (2014) Dancer Perceptions of the Force Reduction of Dance Floors Used by a Professional Touring Ballet Company. *Journal of Dance Medicine and Science*: official publication of the International Association for Dance Medicine & Science **18**(3)

Hubscher, M., Zech, A., Pfeifer, K., Hansel, F., Vogt, L. & Banzer, W. (2010). Neuromuscular training for sports injury prevention: a systematic review. *Medicine and Science in Sports and Exercise*, **42**(3), pp.413–421

Hungerford, B., Gilleard, W. & Hodges, P. (2003). Evidence of altered lumbopelvic muscle recruitment in the presence of sacroiliac joint pain. *Spine*, **28**(14), pp.1593–1600

Hupperets, M., Verhagen, E., Heymans, M., Bosmans, J., van Tulder, M. & van Mechelen, W. (2010). Potential savings of a program to prevent ankle sprain recurrence: economic evaluation of a randomized controlled trial. *American Journal of Sports Medicine*, **38**(11), pp.2194–2200

International Association of Dance Medicine and Science (2009). IADMS. Available at http://www.iadms.org/displaycommon.cfm?an=8

Jacobs, C., Hincapie, C. & Cassidy, J. (2012). Musculoskeletal injuries and pain in dancers. A systematic review update. *Journal of Dance Medicine and Science*, **16**(2), pp.4–84

Jadad, A., Cook, D., Jones, A., Klassen, T., Tugwell, P., Moher, M. & Moher, D. (1998). Methodology and reports of systematic reviews and meta-analyses: a comparison of Cochrane reviews with articles published in paper-based journals. *Journal of the American Medical Association*, **280** pp.278–280

Janda, D. H. (1997). Sports injury surveillance had everything to do with sports medicine. *Sports Medicine*, **24**(3), pp.169–171

Jain, S. & Brown, D. R. (2001). Cultural dance: an opportunity to encourage physical activity and health in communities. *American Journal of Health Education*, **32**(4), pp.216–222

Jones, R. S. and Taggart, T. (1994). Sport-related injuries attending the accident and emergency department. *British Journal of Sports Medicine*, **28**(2), pp.110–111

Jull, G., Trott, P., Potter, H., Zito, G., Niere, K., Shirley, D. et al. (2002). A randomized controlled trial of exercise and manipulative therapy for cervicogenic headache. *Spine*, **27**(17), pp.1835–1843

Kay, T. M., Gross, A., Goldsmith, C. H., Hoving, J. L. & Brønfort, G. Exercises for mechanical neck disorders. *Cochrane Database of Systematic Reviews* 2005, Issue **3**. Art. No.: CD004250. DOI: 10.1002/14651858.CD004250.pub3

Khan, K., Brown, J., Way, S., Vass, N., Crichton, K., Alexander, R., et al. (1995). Overuse injuries in classical ballet. *Sports Medicine*, **19**(5), pp.341–357

Kibler, W. B. Shoulder rehabilitation: principles and practice. *Med Sci Sports Exerc.* 1998 Apr; **30**(4 Suppl):S40–S50. [PubMed]

Kibler, W. B. The role of the scapula in athletic shoulder function. *Am J Sports Med.* 1998 Mar-Apr; **26**(2):325–337. [PubMed]

Kiesel, Plisky & Voight. (2007). Can serious injury in professional football be predicted by a preseason functional movement screen? *North American Journal of Sports Physical Therapy*, **2**(3), pp.147–158

Klemp, P. & Learmonth, I. (1984). Hypermobility and injuries in a professional ballet company. *British Journal of Sports Medicine*, **18**, pp.143–148

Koutedakis, Y., Agrawal, A. & Sharp, N. C. C. (1999). Isokinetic characteristics of knee flexors and extensors in male dancers, Olympic oarsmen, Olympic bobsleighers, and non-athletes. *Journal of Dance Medicine and Science*, **2**(2), pp.63–67

Koutedakis, Y. and Jamurtas, A. (2004). The dancer as a performing athlete: physiological considerations. *Sports Medicine*, **34**(10), pp.651–661

Koutedakis, Y., Stavropoulos-Kalinoglou, A. & Metsios, G. (2005). The Significance of Muscular Strength in Dance. *Journal of Dance Medicine and Science*, **9**(1), pp.29–34

Laws, H. (2005). *Fit to Dance 2 – Report of the second national inquiry into dancers' health and injury in the UK*. London: Newgate Press

Laws, H. (2003). Initial findings of the second national inquiry into dancers' health and injury in the UK: a comparison study. *Journal of Dance Medicine and Science*, **7**(2), pp.62–63

Lee, A. J., Garraway, W. M., Hepburn, W. & Laidlaw, R. (2001). Influence of rugby injuries on players' subsequent health and lifestyle: beginning a long-term follow-up. *British Journal of Sports Medicine*, **35**(1), pp.38–42

Levangie, P. & Norkin, C. (2005) *Joint structure and function: A Comprehensive Analysis*, 4th ed. Philadelphia, PA: F.A. Davis Co. Chicago/Turabian

Liederbach, M. (2010). Perspectives on dance science rehabilitation. Understanding the whole body mechanics and principals of motor control as a basis for healthy movement. *Journal of Dance Medicine and Science*, **14**(3), pp.114–124

Liederbach, M. (1997). Screening for functional capacity in dancers: designing standardized, dance-specific injury prevention screening tools. *Journal of Dance Medicine and Science*, **1**(3), pp.93–106

Liederbach, M. Higgins, Gamboa & J.M. Welsh (2012) Assessing and Reporting Dancer Capacities, Risk Factors, and Injuries: Recommendations from the IADMS Standard Measures Consensus Initiative. *Journal of Dance Medicine and Science*, **16**(4) pp.139–153

Liederbach, M. & Richardson, M. (2007). The importance of standardized injury reporting in dance. *Journal of Dance Medicine and Science*, **11**(2), pp.45–48

Lin, C.C., Delahunt, E. & King, E. (2012). Neuromuscular training for chronic ankle instability. *Physical Therapy*, **92**:987–991

Lippert, L.S. (2011). *Clinical Kinesiology and Anatomy*, 5th ed. Philadelphia, PA: F.A. Davis.

Mansfield, P.J., & Neumann, D.A. (2009). *Essentials of Kinesiology for the Physical Therapist Assistant*. St. Louis, MO: Mosby Elsevier

Ljungqvist, A., Jenoure, P., Engebretsen, L., Alonso, J. M., Bahr, R., Clough, A., De Bondt, G., Dvorak, J., Maloley, R., Matheson, G., Meeuwisse, W., Meijboom, E., Mountjoy, M., Pelliccia, A., Schwellnus, M., Sprumont, D., Schamasch, P., Gauthier, J. B., Dubi, C., Stupp, H. & Thill, C. (2009). The International Olympic Committee (IOC) Consensus Statement on periodic health evaluation of elite athletes March 2009. *British Journal of Sports Medicine*, **43**(9), pp.631–643

Luke, A. C., Kinney, S. A., D'hemecourt, P. A., Baum, J., Owen, M. & Micheli, L. J. (2002). Determinants of injuries in young dancers. *Medical Problems of Performing Artists*, **17**(3), pp.105–112

Lundon, K., Melcher, L. and Bray, K. (1999). Stress fractures in ballet: a twenty-five year review. *Journal of Dance Medicine and Science*, **3**(3), pp.101–107

Macintyre, J. & Joy, E. (2000). Foot and ankle injuries in dance. *Clinics in Sports Medicine*, **19**(2), p.351–368

Manchikanti, L. (2008). Evidence-based medicine, systematic reviews, and guidelines in interventional pain management, part 1: introduction and general considerations. *Pain Physician*, **11**: pp.61–186

Mandelbaum, B., Silvers, H., Watanabe, D., Knarr, J., Thomas, S., Griffin, L., Kirkendall, D. & Garett, W. (2005). Effectiveness of a neuromuscular and proprioceptive training program in preventing anterior cruciate ligament injuries in female athletes. *American Journal of Sports Medicine*. **33**(7), pp.1003–1010

Marshall, P. W., Mannion, J. & Murphy, B. A. (2010). The eccentric, concentric strength relationship of the hamstring muscles in chronic low back pain. *Journal of Electromyography & Kinesiology*, **20**(1), pp.39–45

Masouros, S. D. et al. (2010). *Orthop Trauma*, 2010, **24**: 84–91

McCormack, M., Briggs, J., Hakim, A., & Grahame, R. (2004). Joint laxity and the benign joint hypermobility syndrome in student and professional ballet dancers. *Journal of Rheumatology*, **31**(1), pp.173–178

McGill, S. (2010). Core training: evidence translating to better performance and injury prevention. *Strength and Conditioning Journal*, **32**(3), pp.33–46

Meeuwisse, W. H. (1991). Predictability of sports injuries. What is the epidemiological evidence? *Sports Medicine* (Auckland, NZ), **12**(1), pp.8–15

Meeuwisse, W. H. (1994). Assessing causation in sport injury: a multifactorial model. *Clinical Journal of Sport Medicine*, **4**(3), pp.166–170

Meeuwisse, W. H. & Love, E. J. (1997). Athletic injury reporting: development of universal systems. *Sports Medicine*, **24**(3), pp.184–204

Meeuwisse, W. H., Tyreman, H., Hagel, B. & Emery, C. (2007). A Dynamic Model of Etiology in Sport Injury: The Recursive Nature of Risk and Causation. *Clinical Journal of Sport Medicine*, **17**(3), pp.215–219

Menetrey, J. & Fritschy, D. (1999). Subtalar subluxation in ballet dancers. *American Journal of Sports Medicine*, **27**(2), pp.143–149

Mens, J., Stam, H., Vleeming, A. & Snijders, C. (1995). Active straight-leg raising. A clinical approach to the load transfer function of the pelvic girdle. Rotterdam: ECO.2nd Interdisciplinary World Congress on Low Back Pain, pp.207–220

Milan, K. R. (1994). Injury in ballet: a review of relevant topics for the physical therapist. *Journal of Orthopaedic and Sports Physical Therapy*, **19**(2), pp.121–129

Milan, K. (1996). Literature review of common injuries in the performing artist. *Orthopaedic Physical Therapy Clinics of North America*, **5**(4), pp.421–453

Minick, K. I., Kiesel, K. B., Burton, L., Taylor, A., Plisky, P. & Butler, R. J. (2010). Interrater reliability of the functional movement screen. *Journal of Strength and Conditioning Research*, **24**(2), pp.79–486

Miyamoto, R. G., Dhotar, H. S., Rose, D. J. & Egol, K. (2009). Surgical treatment of refractory tibial stress fractures in elite dancers: a case series. The *American Journal of Sports Medicine*, **37**(6), pp.1150–1154

Moher, D., Liberati, A., Tetzlaff, J., Altman, D. The PRISMA Group (2009). Preferred reporting items for systematic reviews and meta-analysis: The PRISMA statement. *PLoS Med*, **6**(6): e1000097.doi:10.137/journal.pmed 1000097

Moseley, G. & Hodges, P. (2006). Reduced variability of postural strategy prevents normalisation of motor changes induced by back pain: A risk factor for chronic trouble? *Behavioural Neuroscience*, **120**(2), pp.474–476

Mottram, S. & Comerford, M. (2008). A new perspective on risk assessment. *Physical Therapy in Sport*, **9**(1), pp.40–51

Murphy, D. F., Connolly, D. A. J. & Beynnon, B. D. (2003). Risk factors for lower extremity injury: a review of the literature. *British Journal of Sports Medicine*, **37**(1), pp.13–29

Myer, G., Ford, K., Palumbo, J. & Hewett, T. (2005). Neuromuscular training improves performance and lower extremity biomechanics in female athletes. *Journal of Strength and Conditioning Research*, **19**(1), pp.51–60

Myklebust, G. & Bahr, R. (2005). Return to play guidelines after anterior cruciate ligament surgery. *British Journal of Sports Medicine*, **39**(3), pp.127–131

Nordin, M. & Frankel, V. (2012) Basic biomechanics of the musculoskeletal system. Lippincott Williams and Wilkins

Nilsson, C., Leanderson, J., Wykman, A. & Strender, L. E. (2001). The injury panorama in a Swedish professional ballet company. *Knee Surgery, Sports Traumatology, Arthroscopy,* **9**(4), pp.242–246

Noyes, F. R., Barber, S. D. & Mangine, R. E. Abnormal lower limb symmetry determined by function hop tests after anterior cruciate ligament rupture. *Am J Sports Med*, **19**:513–8

O'Conner, F., Deuster, P., Davis, J., Pappas, C. & Knapik, J. (2011). Functional movement screening: Predicting injuries in officer candidates. *Medicine and Science in Sports and Exercise*. Vol. **43**, No. 12, pp.224–2230

O'Driscoll, J. & Delahunt, E. (2011). Neuromuscular training to enhance sensorimotor and functional deficits in subjects with chronic ankle instability: a systematic review and best evidence synthesis. *Sports Medicine, Arthroscopy, Rehabilitation, Therapy and Technology,* **3**:19

O'Mailia, S. P., Scharff-Olson, M. & Williford, H. N. (2002). Activity monitors and dance-based exercise: estimating caloric expenditure. *Journal of Dance Medicine and Science*, **6**(2), pp.50–53

Orchard, J. & Hoskins, W. (2007). For debate: consensus injury definitions in team sports should focus on missed playing time. *Clinical Journal of Sport Medicine*, **17**(3), pp.192–196

Onate, J., Dewey, T., Kollock, R., Thomas, K., Van Lunen, B., DeMaio, M. & Ringler, S. (2012). Real-time intersession and interrater reliability of the functional movement screen. *Journal of Strength and Conditioning Research*. **26**(2):408–415

O'Sullivan, P. (2005). Diagnosis and classification of chronic low back pain disorders: Maladaptive movement and motor control impairments as underlying mechanisms. *Manual Therapy*, **10**(4), pp.242–255

O'Sullivan, P. (2000). Lumbar segmental 'instability' clinical presentation and specific stabilizing exercise management. *Manual Therapy*, **5**(1), pp.2–12

O'Sullivan, P., Twomey, L. & Allison, G. (1997). Evaluation of specific stabilisation exercise in the treatment of chronic low back pain with a radiological diagnosis of spondylosis or spondylolisthesis. *Spine*, **22**(24), pp.2959–2967

Parkkari, J., Kujala, U. M. & Kannus, P. (2001). Is it possible to prevent sports injuries? Review of controlled clinical trials and recommendations for future work. *Sports Medicine*, **31**(14), pp.985–995

Peate, Bates, Lunda, Francis & Bellamy. (2007). Core strength: A new model for injury prediction and prevention. *Journal of Occupational Medicine and Toxicology*, **2**(3), pp.1–9

Pedersen, M. E. & Wilmerding, V. (1998). Injury profiles of student and professional flamenco dancers. *Journal of Dance Medicine and Science*, **2**(3), pp.108–114

Penrod, J. (1994). Expression in dance: teaching beyond technique. *Impulse*, **2**, pp.3–15

Peterson, M., Rhea, M. & Alvar, B. (2005). Applications of the dose response for muscular development: a review of meta-analytic efficiency and reliability for designing training prescription. *Journal of Strength and Conditioning Research*, **19**(4), pp.950–958

Phillips, H. (2000) Sports injury incidence. *British Journal of Sports Medicine*, **34**, pp.133–136

Pluim, B. M., Fuller, C. W., Batt, M. E., Chase, L., Hainline, B., Miller, S. et al. (2009). Consensus statement on epidemiological studies of medical conditions in tennis, April 2009. *British Journal of Sports Medicine*, **43**(12), pp.893–897

Prisk, V., O'Loughlin, P. & Kennedy, J. (2008). Forefoot injuries in dancers. *Clinics in Sports Medicine*, **27**(2), pp.305–320

Pollock et al. (2014) British Athletics muscle injury classification: a new grading system. *BJSM*, **48**, pp.1347–1351

Pool-Goudzwaard, A. L., Vleeming, A., Stoeckart, R., Snijders, C. J. & Mens, J. M. (1998). Insufficient lumbopelvic stability: a clinical, anatomical and biomechanical approach to 'a-specific' low back pain. *Manual Therapy*, **3**(1), pp.12–20

Quirk, R. (1983). Ballet injuries: the Australian experience. *Clinics in Sports Medicine*, **2**(3), pp.507–514

Ramal, E. & Moritz, U. (1994). Self reported musculoskeletal pain and discomfort in professional ballet dancers in Sweden. *Scandinavian Journal of Rehabilitation Medicine*, **26**(1), pp.11–16

Ramal, E., Moritz, U. & Jarnlo, G. (1996). Recurrent musculo-skeletal pain in professional ballet dancers in Sweden: A six-year follow up. *Journal of Dance Medicine and Science*, **3**(3), pp.93–100

Rambaud, A. J. M. et al. (2017) Criteria for Return to Sport after Anterior Cruciate Ligament reconstruction with lower reinjury risk (CR'STAL study): protocol for a prospective observational study in France BMJ Open, 7:e015087.doi:10.1136/bmjopen–2016–015087

Russell, B. (1991). A study of lumbopelvic dysfunction/psoas insufficiency and its role as a major cause of dance injury. *Chiropractic Sports Medicine*, **5**(1), pp.9–17

Russell, Shave, Yoshioka, Kruse, Koutedakis & Wyon (2010). Magnetic resonance imaging of the ankle in female ballet dancers en pointe. *Acta Radiologica*, *51*(6), pp.655–661

Schulz, K., Altman, D. & Moher, D. (2010) CONSORT 2010 Statement: updated guidelines for reporting parallel group randomised trials. *British Medical Journal*, **340**: 698–702

Scott, G. (1997). Banes and Carroll on defining dance. *Dance Research Journal*, **29**(1), pp.7–23

Schon, L., Biddinger, K., Greenwood, P. (1994). Dance screen programs and development of dance clinics. *Clinics in Sports Medicine*, **13**(4), pp.865–882

Shah, S. (2008). Caring for the dancer: Special considerations for the performer and troupe. *Current Sports Medicine Reports*, **7**(3), pp.28–132

Shea, B., Grimshaw, J., Wells, G., Boers, M., Andersson, N., Hamel, C., Porter, A., Tugwell, P., Moher, D. & Bouter, L. (2007) Development of AMSTAR: a measurement tool to assess the methodological quality of systematic reviews. *BMC Medical Research Methodology*, 7:10 doi10.1186/1471–2288–7–10

Shrier, I., Meeuwisse, W. H., Matheson, G. O., Wingfield, K., Steele, R. J., Prince, F. et al. (2009). Injury Patterns and Injury Rates in the Circus Arts: An Analysis of 5 Years of Data From Cirque du Soleil. *American Journal of Sports Medicine*, **37**(6), pp.1143–1149

Siev-Ner, I., Barak, A., Heim, M., Warshavsky, M. & Azaria, M. (1997). The value of screening. *Journal of Dance Medicine and Science*, **1**(3), pp.87–92

Snijders, C. Vleeming, A. & Stoeckart, R. (1993). Transfer of lumbosacral load to the iliac bones and legs. Part 1: biomechanics of self-bracing of the sacroiliac joints and its significance for treatment and exercise. *Clinical Biomechanics*, **8**, pp.285–294

Sohl, P. and Bowling, A. (1990). Injuries to dancers : prevalence, treatment and prevention. *Patient Management*, **14**(9), pp.69–75;95

Solomon, R., Micheli, L., Solomon, J. & Kelley, T. (1995). The cost of injuries in a professional ballet company: Anatomy of a season. *Medical Problems of Performing Artists*, **10**(1), pp.3–10

Solomon, R., Micheli, L., Solomon, J. & Kelley, T. (1996). The cost of injuries in a professional ballet company: A three-year perspective. *Medical problems of performing artists*, **11**(3), pp.67–74

Solomon, R., Solomon, J., Micheli, J. & McGray, E. (1999). The cost of injuries in a professional ballet company: A five-year study. *Medical Problems of Performing Artists*, **14**(4), pp.164–169

Sommer, H. M. & Vallentyne, S. W. (1995). Effect of foot posture on the incidence of medial tibial stress syndrome/Effet de la posture du pied sur la frequence d'apparition du syndrome de stress median tibial. *Medicine & Science in Sports & Exercise*, **27**(6), pp.800–804

Southwick, H. & Cassella, M. (2002). Boston Ballet student screening clinic: an aid to injury prevention. *Orthopaedic Physical Therapy Practice*, **14**(2), pp.14–16

Stretanski, M. (2002). Classical ballet: the full contact sport. *American Journal of Physical Medicine Rehabilitation*, **81**, pp.392–393

Stroup, D., Berlin, J., Morton, S., Olkin, S., Williamson, G., Rennie, D., Moher, D., Becker, B., Sipe, T. & Thacker, S. (2000). Meta-analysis of observational studies in epidemiology. *Journal of the American Medical Association*, **19**, 283, pp.5208–2012

Teitz, C. C., & Kilcoyne, R. F. (1998). Premature osteoarthrosis in professional dancers. *Clinical Journal of Sport Medicine*: *Official Journal Of The Canadian Academy Of Sport Medicine*, 8(4), pp.255–259

Tenforde, A. Shull, P. & Fredericson, M. (2012). Neuromuscular prehabilitation to prevent osteoarthritis after traumatic joint injury. *Physical Medicine and Rehabilitation*, **4**:s141–s144

Teyhen, D., Shaffer, S., Lorenson, C., Halfpap, J., Donofry, D., Walker, M., Dugan, J. & Childs, J. (2012). The functional movement screen: a reliability study. *Journal of Orthopaedics and Sports Physical Therapy*, **42**(6), pp.530–540

Trees, A. H., Howe, T. E., Grant, M., & Gray, H. G. Exercise for treating anterior cruciate ligament injuries in combination with collateral ligament and meniscal damage of the knee in adults. *Cochrane Database of Systematic Reviews* 2007, Issue **3**. Art. No.: CD005961. DOI: 10.1002/14651858.CD005961.pub2

Trees, A. H., Howe, T. E., Dixon, J., & White, L. Exercise for treating isolated anterior cruciate ligament injuries in adults. *Cochrane Database of Systematic Reviews* 2005, Issue **4**. Art. No.: CD005316. DOI: 10.1002/14651858.CD005316.pub2

Trojian, T., McKeag, D. (2006) Single-leg balance test to identify risk of ankle sprains. *British Journal of Sports Medicine*, **40**(7), pp.610–613

Twitchett, E., Angioi, M., Koutedakis, Y. et al. (2010). The demands of a working day among female professional ballet dancers. *Journal of Dance Medicine and Science*, **4**, pp.127–132

Twitchett, E., Angioi, M., Koutedakis, Y. & Wyon, M. (2009). Video Analysis of Classical Ballet Performance. *Journal of Dance Medicine and Science*, **13**(4), pp.124–128

van Dijk, C. Lim, Poortman, A. Strubbe, E. & Marti, R. (1995). Degenerative joint disease in female ballet dancers. *American Journal of Sports Medicine*, **23**(3), pp:295–300

van Mechelen, W., Hlobil, H. & Kemper, H. C. G. (1992). Incidence, severity, aetiology and prevention of sports injuries: a review of concepts/Incidence, gravité, etiologie et prevention des traumatismes sportifs: une revue de concepts). *Sports Medicine*, **14**(2), pp.82–99

Vann, M. A. & Manoli, A. (2010). Medial Ankle Impingement Syndrome in Female Gymnasts. *Operative Techniques in Sports Medicine*, **18**(1), pp.50–52

Verhagen, E. & Bay, K. (2010). Optimising ankle sprain prevention: a critical review and practical appraisal of the literature. *British Journal of Sports Medicine*. **44**:1082–1088

Wainner, R. S., Whitman, J. M., Cleland, J. A. & Flynn, T. W. (2007). Regional interdependence: a musculoskeletal examination model whose time has come. *Journal of Orthopaedic and Sports Physical Therapy*, **37**(11), pp.658–660

Warren, M., Brooks-Gunn, J., Hamilton, L., Warren, L. & Hamilton, W. (1986). Scoliosis and fractures in young ballet dancers. Relation to delayed menarche and secondary amenorrhea. *New England Journal of Medicine*, **314**(21), pp.1348–1353

Wheeler, L. P. (1987). Common musculoskeletal dance injuries. *Chiropractic Sports Medicine*, **1**(1), pp:17–23

White and Panjabi (1990) *Clinical Biomechanics of the Spine*, 2nd Edition. J P Lippincott Company

Wiesler, E. R., Hunter, M., Martin, D., Curl, W. W. & Hoen, H. (1996) Ankle flexibility and injury patterns in dancers. *American Journal of Sports Medicine*, **24**(6), pp.754–757

Willson, J. Dougherty, C. Ireland, M. & Davis, I (2005). Core stability and its relationship to lower extremity function and injury. *Journal of the American Academy of Orthopaedic Surgeons*, **13**(5), pp.316–25

Wingfield, K., Matheson, G. & Meeuwisse, W. (2004). Preparticipation evaluation: an evidence-based review. *Clinical Journal of Sports Medicine*, **14**, pp.109–122

Wolman, R. & Allen, N. (2013). Vitamin D status in professional ballet dancers: Winter vs. summer. DOI:10.1016/j.jsams.2012.12.010

Wyon. M., Allen, N. et al. (2006) Anthropometric factors affecting jump height in ballet dancers. Journal of *Dance Medicine and Science* January 2006, **10**(3&4) pp.106–110

Wyon, M. & Allen, N (2007) The Cardiorespiratory, Anthropometric, and Performance Characteristics of an International/National Touring Ballet Company. *Journal of Strength and Conditioning Research.* **21**(2), pp.389–93

Wyon, M. & Allen, N. (2013) The influence of winter vitamin D supplementation on muscle function and injury occurrence in elite ballet dancers: A controlled study DOI:10.1016/j.jsams.2013.03.007

Wyon, M., Head, A., Sharp, N. C. C., Redding, E. & Abt, G. (2004). Oxygen Uptake During Modern Dance Class, Rehearsal, and Performance. *Journal of Strength and Conditioning Research*, **18**(3), pp.646–649

Wyon, M. & Reading, E. (2005). Physiological Monitoring of Cardiorespiratory Adaptations During Rehearsal and Performance of Contemporary Dance. *Journal of Strength and Conditioning Research.* **19**(3), pp.611–614

Wyon, M. Twitchet, E. et al. (2011). Time Motion and Video Analysis of Classical Ballet and Contemporary Dance Performance. *International Journal of Sports Medicine*, **32**(11), pp.851–5

Yates, B. & White, S. (2004). The incidence and risk factors in the development of medial tibial stress syndrome among naval recruits. *American Journal of Sports Medicine*, **32**(3), pp.772–780

Yoo, J., Lim, B., Ha, M., Lee, S., Oh, S., Lee, Y. & Kim, J. (2010). A meta-analysis of the effect of neuromuscular training on the prevention of the anterior cruciate ligament injury in female athletes. *Knee Surg Sports Traumatol Athrosc.* **18**, pp.824–830

Zech, A., Hubscher, M., Vogt, L., Banzer, W., Hansel, F. & Pfeifer, K. (2010). Balance training for neuromuscular control and performance enhancement: a systematic review. *Journal of Athletic Training.* **45**(40), pp.392–403

Zöch, C., Fialka-Moser, V. & Quittan, M. (2003). Rehabilitation of ligamentous ankle injuries: a review of recent studies. *British Journal of Sports Medicine*, **37**(4), pp.291–295

INDEX